STAFFING
THE
MEDICAL
PRACTICE

DEBORAH WALKER KEEGAN
PhD, FACMPE
ELIZABETH WALLACE WOODCOCK
MBA, FACMPE, CPC

STAFFING
THE
MEDICAL
PRACTICE

DEBORAH WALKER KEEGAN
PhD, FACMPE
ELIZABETH WALLACE WOODCOCK
MBA, FACMPE, CPC

MGMA
Medical Group Management Association

Medical Group Management Association© (MGMA©) publications are intended to provide current and accurate information and are designed to assist readers in becoming more familiar with the subject matter covered. Such publications are distributed with the understanding that MGMA does not render any legal, accounting, or other professional advice that may be construed as specifically applicable to individual situations. No representations or warranties are made concerning the application of legal or other principles discussed by the authors to any specific factual situation, nor is any prediction made concerning how any particular judge, government official, or other person will interpret or apply such principles. Specific factual situations should be discussed with professional advisors.

Production Credits
Senior Product Manager: Craig Wiberg, MLS, MBA
Content Production Editor: Keith J Olexa
Page Design, Composition, and Production: EGZ Publications

Library of Congress Cataloging-in-Publication Data
Names: Keegan, Deborah Walker, author. | Woodcock, Elizabeth W., author.
Title: Staffing the medical practice / Deborah Walker Keegan, Elizabeth
  Wallace Woodcock.
Description: [Englewood, Colorado] : Medical Group Management Association,
  [2018] | Includes bibliographical references and index.
Identifiers: LCCN 2018042902 (print) | LCCN 2018043859 (ebook) | ISBN
  9781568295473 (e-book) | ISBN 9781568295466 (pbk.)
Subjects: | MESH: Practice Management, Medical--organization & administration
  | Personnel Staffing and Scheduling--organization & administration
Classification: LCC R728 (ebook) | LCC R728 (print) | NLM W 80 | DDC
  610.68--dc23
p. ; cm.
Summary: "Staffing tools and techniques to help medical practice administrators create the 'right' care team for their medical practice--one that is current with today's delivery system and that optimizes provider productivity and efficiency, practice profitability, staff recruitment and retention, and patient value"--Provided by publisher. 1. Medical offices--Management. I. Medical Group Management Association. II. Title. [DNLM: 1. Office Management--organization & administration. 2. Practice Management, Medical--organization & administration. W 80 W886f 2011]

Item: 9158
ISBN: 978-1-56829-546-6

Printed in the United States of America 10 9 8 7 6 5 4 3 2 1

DEDICATION

This book is dedicated to our friend and colleague
Marc A. West.
An extraordinary leader who empowers others with his courage and
expertise to be their best selves.

Acknowledgements

We extend our appreciation to the many physicians, advanced practice providers, hospital and system leaders, medical practice executives and practice site and business office employees with whom we have worked and those who have attended our seminars. You continue to educate and stimulate us to critical thought. Thank you for your commitment, dedication and the exceptional efforts you make on behalf of your practices and the patients you serve.

TABLE OF CONTENTS

INTRODUCTION

We are witnessing a transformation of medical practice staffing, from a narrow focus on staffing the provider to care team models involved in key elements of patient-facing visits and remote care. There are new patient access channels, new care delivery systems, new value-based payment models, and new patient population management strategies. Each requires novel knowledge and skills, and all of which impact the staffing deployment model you adopt for your medical practice. Changes to staffing models—to align the medical practice with today's healthcare environment—are presented throughout this book.

In Part 1 of this book, we discuss the importance of correctly staffing the medical practice.

- In Chapter 1: Impact of Staffing on the Medical Practice, we report the positive impacts of appropriate staffing and the negative impacts of inappropriate staffing on a medical practice.
- In Chapter 2: How Staffing Affects Practice Profitability and Performance, via staff data and regression analyses, we demonstrate the important relationships between staffing, profitability, and performance so you can leverage this in your medical practice.

In Part 2 of the book, we share two methods to identify whether your practice has the right number and right skill mix of staff on your care team.

- In Chapter 3: Staff Benchmarking, we describe how to compare your current staffing with benchmark data related to the number of staff, the skill mix of staff, and the cost of staff in your medical practice.
- In Chapter 4: Staff Productivity, we help you analyze the current productivity of your staff and compare it with expected staff productivity ranges to determine if you have staffing opportunity.

We detail how to staff key patient flow and business processes in a medical practice in Part 3. We utilize the benchmarking and productivity tools to "build" the optimal staffing models for each of the key patient flow processes in the medical practice, to include:

- Chapter 5: Staffing Communications

- Chapter 6: Staffing the Front Office
- Chapter 7: Staffing the Encounter
- Chapter 8: Staffing the Business Office
- Chapter 9: Staffing for Value-Based Care

Part 4 is devoted to optimizing your staffing deployment model.

- In Chapter 10: Staffing Deployment Models, we share methods to analyze your staffing deployment model and look for areas of opportunity to redesign the model for optimal performance. Your staffing model has a direct impact on the volume and type of employees needed in your practice. Importantly, the staffing model in a medical practice must change over time to align with the volume and type of work to be performed. We provide tools to help you determine if your staffing model is optimized for future success.

- In Chapter 11: Teleworking and Flexible Staffing, we recognize that today's medical practice needs to be flexible and agile. We discuss teleworking, a win-win strategy for a medical practice and its employees. Technology permits work that is non-patient-facing to be performed remotely, with steps taken to ensure inclusion of these staff in the care team. In Chapter 11, we also discuss part-time, per diem and contract workers to match staff to the actual work that needs to be performed, particularly when there are fluctuating work levels in a medical practice.

And in Part 5 of the book, we share strategies to create a high-performing care team.

- In Chapter 12: High-Performing Care Teams, we share expected teamwork behaviors and management techniques to elevate teamwork in the practice.

- In Chapter 13: Staff Recruitment, Retention and Talent Management, we discuss effective staff recruitment, retention, and performance management techniques.

Throughout this book, we share tools and strategies to help you design an optimal staffing deployment model for your medical practice to ensure value-based care, provider productivity and efficiency, practice profitability, effective staff recruitment and retention, and stellar patient experience and value.

PART 1

IMPORTANCE OF CORRECTLY STAFFING THE MEDICAL PRACTICE

CHAPTER 1

IMPACT OF STAFFING ON THE MEDICAL PRACTICE

Sweeping changes in healthcare are directly impacting the staffing model of today's medical practices. From value-based reimbursement to value-based care, from traditional patient-facing visits to secure messaging and telemedicine, from a focus on individual, personal care to patient population management, we are witnessing fundamental changes that require new staff roles and staffing strategies. Today's medical practice must align its staffing model to effectively compete in a value-based world.

In this chapter, we discuss:

- Effects of appropriate staffing levels
- Consequences of inappropriate skill mix
- Driving forces for staffing innovation

POSITIVE EFFECTS OF APPROPRIATE STAFFING

Staff are instrumental in ensuring quality clinical care; they are the conduit by which patients access their care. If we staff the medical practice correctly, these staff can work in a coordinated and cohesive fashion to ensure that provider and patient needs are met, thereby streamlining the patient flow process. Correctly staffing the medical practice results in optimized patient care and service.

Data suggest that appropriate staffing for a medical practice permits physicians and advanced practice providers to optimize their productivity and efficiency. This is not trivial. The chief constraint in a medical practice is the provider's time. If there are any openings that appear in the schedule — due to a patient failing to keep his or her appointment, for example — that time is gone; it cannot be inventoried.[1]

Though some staff are assigned to directly support the physician to provide clinical services, many functions carried out by the staff in a medical practice are administrative. Indeed, the only truly value-added steps in the entire patient flow process from the patient's point of view is the actual time the patient spends in the exam room with the provider or when receiving remote care, for example, receiving clinical information and instruction via telephone or secure electronic message, or via a telemedicine-based encounter.

Medical practices that are appropriately staffed achieve four key advantages:

- Provider time is optimized. Tasks are delegated to the appropriate staff member based on work type and licensure, resulting is less wasted time.

- Providers can focus on clinical care. Providers effectively use their distinct competencies to evaluate, diagnose, and treat patients and perform the critical tasks necessary to ensure value-based care, reducing administrative tasks and wasted time.

- Patients' satisfaction with key components of their experience is met or exceeded. They perceive a 'patient-first' mission.

- The business of medicine is well-managed. Staff are educated and deployed to the critical business functions required in today's healthcare reimbursement environment.

> INDEED, THE ONLY TRULY VALUE-ADDED STEPS IN THE ENTIRE PATIENT FLOW PROCESS FROM THE PATIENT'S POINT OF VIEW IS THE ACTUAL TIME THE PATIENT SPENDS IN THE EXAM ROOM WITH THE PROVIDER OR WHEN RECEIVING REMOTE CARE.

NEGATIVE EFFECTS OF INAPPROPRIATE STAFFING

Negative consequences can result if your medical practice has either too few or too many staff members.

An insufficient volume of staff to carry out the work may produce the following negative consequences for a medical practice.

LOW PHYSICIAN PRODUCTIVITY

In medical practices with too few staff, physicians are often required to perform non-clinical, administrative tasks. Because no one is there to take on the task, work that would normally be assigned to others is not delegated. This leads to a domino effect: declining physician productivity negatively impacts patient access and, in turn, adversely influences the financial viability of the practice. When there is insufficient staff to manage the work inherent in ambulatory care, exam-room turnover slows and visit assistance diminishes. Consequently, the ratio of new patients to return patients declines, leading to delays in patient access, and for some, closing the practice to new patients, simply because there is insufficient infrastructure.

Problematic Staff Recruitment and Retention

Prospective employees are not keen to work in a medical practice where staff are overextended and overstressed, which is typically the case in medical practices that are under-resourced. Similarly, current employees — often your best and brightest — are asked to perform tasks below their licensure and/or skill level. These stellar employees can recognize that there are jobs outside your practice where their talent and expertise can be used in more meaningful ways, and might be more compelled to seek them out.

Poor Customer Experience

Overextended staff members are often incapable of providing a consistent level of service and support to the patient, let alone the physician. Consequently, the experience of patients, families, as well as referring physicians, declines and can deteriorate to levels where patients no longer want to be seen by your physicians. Customer experience is often considered a proxy for quality. Thus, if service is suboptimal, patients will often interpret this to mean that quality, too, is below par.

Increased Business Risk

Staff may routinely perform tasks that are not consistent with their training and licensure in medical practices with too few staff. For example, a medical assistant starts to resemble a licensed nurse by inappropriately providing clinical advice to the patient. Routinely executing skills that are well below a staff member's training and licensure is problematic as well. Consider an advanced practice provider who is performing tasks, such as triaging telephone calls and rooming patients, that can be appropriately managed by a licensed nurse or medical assistant.

In addition to performing "out of class" assignments, when there are too few staff we often witness work falling through the cracks. Staff just don't have time to address certain key functions, such as reaching out to a no-show patient to determine why he or she missed the appointment and rescheduling that patient for needed care, tracking down a missing test result, or following up on an alert that a patient was just discharged from the hospital. Business risk increases and quality and safety can be compromised by staffing at an inappropriate level.

LACK OF ACCOUNTABILITY

Lack of accountability is also a result of having suboptimal staffing levels. In some practices, staff members are basically assigned to all tasks, with the expectation that they will get to each task when they can. This results in loss of accountability and work discipline. Tasks are often not completed, and when they are, they may be of inconsistent quality.

INABILITY TO MANAGE POPULATION HEALTH

A final consequence of too few staff is failure to address the needs of the patient population outside of the office, instead focusing solely on those patients who present for face-to-face encounters. Lacking the ability to maintain engagement with its entire population of patients, the practice fails to maintain high-quality scores for preventive and recommended follow-up care. Communication with patients between their in-office visits is limited (or nonexistent), and transitions of care are not effectively managed. Instead, patients are often left to self-manage their own course of care, with the practice having only adequate resources to manage patients while physically present in the office setting.

> SERVICE IS OFTEN CONSIDERED A PROXY FOR QUALITY. THUS, IF SERVICE IS SUBOPTIMAL, PATIENTS WILL OFTEN INTERPRET THIS TO MEAN THAT QUALITY, TOO, IS BELOW PAR.

On the other end of the continuum, too many staff at work in a medical practice can also lead to negative consequences, including the following.

HIGH STAFF COST

When there are too many staff, there is commonly low staff productivity, yet staffing costs (and therefore overhead costs) are higher than peer practices, negatively impacting the profitability of the medical practice and the ability to effectively compete for patients or hire new physicians. In these medical practices, the cost of staff as a percentage of total medical revenue is higher than benchmark norms.

As shown in Exhibit 1.1, the cost of staff for most medical practices can exceed 25 percent of total medical revenue generated by the medical practice. This is an expense surpassed only by provider cost.

EXHIBIT 1.1 TOTAL SUPPORT STAFF EXPENSES AS A PERCENTAGE OF TOTAL MEDICAL REVENUE BY PRACTICE SPECIALTY[2]

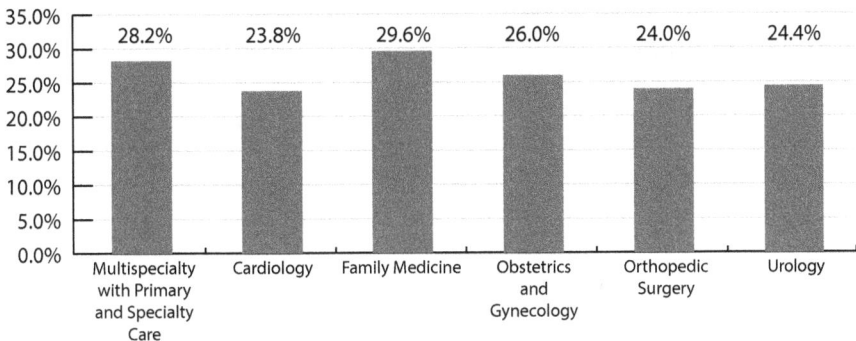

	Multispecialty with Primary and Specialty Care	Cardiology	Family Medicine	Obstetrics and Gynecology	Orthopedic Surgery	Urology
	28.2%	23.8%	29.6%	26.0%	24.0%	24.4%

MGMA DataDive for Cost and Revenue 2017 Report Based on 2016 Data. Copyright MGMA. Reprinted with permission.

It is imperative for a medical practice to staff correctly, to identify the right staff and ask them to perform the right activities to optimize practice efficiency and profitability, and to ensure patients receive quality care and service.

INAPPROPRIATE WORK SCOPE

A second consequence of too many staff is the missing link between staff and the work. The low levels of staff productivity become ingrained into the staff mindset; efforts to increase productivity may be met with resistance and entrenchment. The staff are accustomed to working at a certain tempo; when more is expected, the pace cannot be realistically sustained and staff productivity per unit of work declines. One of the toughest challenges for any medical practice is to intensify productivity once staff are used to working at a certain (often slower) pace.

INCREASE IN HUMAN RESOURCES CHALLENGES

In medical practices with too many staff, employees may have too much time on their hands. With excess downtime, inappropriate activities or behavior may flourish (for example, excessive use of social media and/or gossip). Medical practices with too many staff may experience more human resources challenges than medical practices that have managed to staff correctly.

MORAL HAZARD

In medical practices with high staff volumes, we often see shirking behavior from some staff who do not participate as equal members of the care team. A type of moral hazard, shirking can have a negative impact on collegiality, and the ability to retain high-performing team members.

> ONE OF THE TOUGHEST CHALLENGES FOR ANY MEDICAL PRACTICE IS TO INTENSIFY PRODUCTIVITY ONCE STAFF ARE USED TO WORKING AT A CERTAIN PACE.

CONSEQUENCES OF INAPPROPRIATE SKILL MIX

When an incorrect skill mix or licensure of staff is deployed, the practice suffers. Many of the negative consequences that result when medical practices have too few or too many staff members also apply when there is an improper skill mix of staff. For example, staff may perform out of class. This is a costly staffing model in which licensed staff perform routine tasks that can be delegated to other, less qualified staff or, alternatively, when staff are asked to perform work that is beyond their level of competency. This can lead to business risk in a medical practice, negatively impacting patient safety, quality of care, and patient experience. It can also result in a high-cost staffing model and inappropriate support for the provider.

As this discussion demonstrates, the staff in a medical practice play a vital role in its success. The impact of incorrect staffing is detrimental to the medical practice, negatively impacting patient care and safety, staff recruitment and retention, medical practice productivity and profitability, and customer experience. The consequences of inappropriate staffing of a medical practice are summarized in Exhibit 1.2.

EXHIBIT 1.2 CONSEQUENCES OF INAPPROPRIATE STAFFING

Too Few Staff	• Low physician productivity • Problematic recruitment and retention • Poor customer experience • Increased business risk • Lack of accountability • Inability to manage population health
Too Many Staff	• High staff cost • Inappropriate work scope • More human resources challenges • Moral hazard
Inappropriate Skill Mix of Staff	• Increased business risk • High cost • Inappropriate work scope • Low physician productivity • Poor customer experience

DRIVING FORCES FOR STAFFING INNOVATION

Medical practices are increasingly embracing innovative staffing models and strategies in part due to the following:

TRANSITION TO VALUE-BASED CARE

Staffing models have been altered to align with value-based reimbursement. As an example, today's medical practice staff must be deployed to manage point of care collections due to high deductible health plans. Similarly, clinical staff are now deployed to manage the quality and cost of care and to perform new roles due to expanded patient access channels, care outreach, and patient engagement as part of personal, value-based care delivery models.

TECHNOLOGY INNOVATION

New technologies permit medical practices to deliver care outside of the traditional patient-facing visit. Staff are learning new skills and are being delegated new roles and responsibilities for remote care and expanded care team engagement.

PATIENT FLOW REDESIGN

Many practices are redesigning their patient flow process to improve service to patients. As an example, some medical practices have eliminated the need for patients to travel to a check-in or check-out area by instead conducting this work either pre-visit or in the exam room. Patient flow redesign is accompanied by staffing model redesign to ensure alignment.

RECRUITMENT AND RETENTION OF HIGH PERFORMERS

Many practices are now focusing efforts on their high performers, some of whom may be offered flexible work hours or teleworking opportunities. Similarly, today's employees are expected to contribute their knowledge and expertise to the medical practice to assist with change efforts and ensure competitive advantage.

In today's medical practices, we need to deploy the staff and harness their talents and contributions to optimally support four patient flow processes: (1) communications, (2) front office, (3) encounter and (4) value-based care (see Exhibit 1.3). Note that these are in addition to staffing the requisite business of medicine processes, to include the revenue cycle. In this book, we have dedicated chapters to each of these processes.

- *The communication process.* The communication process involves the channels used by patients to contact a practice for both clinical and business communications — to schedule an appointment, obtain an answer to a clinical question, ask questions regarding a bill, obtain laboratory test results, and a host of other issues. Whether using a registry, portal, or smart phone, these methods of communication and access need to be supported by qualified staff.

- *The front office process.* Today's front office is complex. Patient financial clearance, reception and check-in, check-out and referral management require staff to master new knowledge and skills as they serve as the visible representation of your medical practice. Staff must learn how to support new technologies, to include self-serve technologies, such as patient self-registration, self-scheduling, and secure messaging.

- *The encounter process.* This process involves the work that occurs during a face-to-face visit with a patient, including patient reception and arrival, patient retrieval, rooming and intake, the encounter itself, and patient discharge from the exam room. Importantly, clinical support staff must now support the patient portal and remote care; clinical staff roles are changing due to electronic health record (EHR) systems and value-based care requirements.

- *The value-based care process.* Management of today's patient is essentially individual population management. Patients expect personalized care and access to care and information on a 24/7 basis. This requires staffing models for new patient access channels and new value-added services, with staff deployed to manage care outreach, transitions of care, panel and population health management, health coaching, secure messaging, data analytics, and business intelligence. Care teams are engaging patients to partner with them to meet patients' personal care needs.

> IN ADDITION TO TRADITIONAL FLOW PROCESSES, THE PORTAL, VIDEO VISITS, PANEL MANAGEMENT, HEALTH COACHING, CARE OUTREACH, SECURE MESSAGING, AND REMOTE CARE REQUIRE A DISTINCT FOCUS OF STAFF ROLES AND RESPONSIBILITIES.

Importantly, today's medical practice employs multiple technologies to conduct each of these patient flow processes. For example:

- A visit with the patient's physician may involve a face-to-face visit, a visit via telephone or video or via secure messaging with the physician.

- The visit may be initiated by patient request via the telephone or secure messaging, via a remote technology alert from the patient's mobile device, or via a nurse working the patient registry and recognizing outstanding care needs.
- The location of the visit may be at the medical practice or at the patient's home or work site.

The care team must be aligned to support each of these delivery systems as we transition to value-based care. We need the right staff performing the right activities so that we can provide the right care in the right setting at the right cost for patients.

EXHIBIT 1.3 STAFFING FOR FOUR PATIENT FLOW PROCESSES

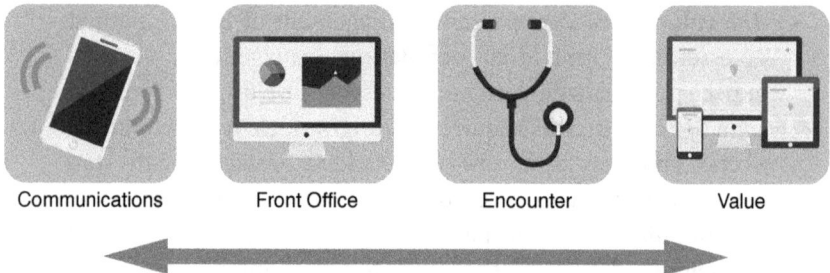

| Communications | Front Office | Encounter | Value |

SUMMARY

A medical practice that simply reduces staff is not going to achieve long-term, sustainable financial performance. Why? When staff are cut below the level necessary to run an effective and efficient practice, there is waste. One key category of that waste is physicians being asked to perform nonclinical tasks. As we discuss in this chapter, it is vital for a medical practice to staff correctly — to assemble the appropriate number of staff with the right skill mix — to provide appropriate infrastructure and support to the provider and to achieve optimal physician productivity, practice profitability, and patient experience.

ENDNOTES

1 A detailed discussion of this concept can be found in Woodcock, Elizabeth W. 2014. Mastering Patient Flow: 4th Edition. Englewood, Colo.: Medical Group Management Association.

2 MGMA DataDive for Cost and Revenue 2017 Report Based on 2016 Data. Copyright MGMA. Reprinted with permission.

CHAPTER 2

HOW STAFFING AFFECTS PRACTICE PRODUCTIVITY AND PERFORMANCE

Guest Co-Author: David N. Gans

By analyzing staffing data and the relationship between data elements, we learn insights on how best to staff a medical practice. Staffing data, to include the number of staff, skill mix of staff, and cost of staff, are available at the specialty level for most medical and surgical disciplines. From these data, we learn important lessons to help practices staff for optimal performance.

In this chapter, we discuss:

- Staffing by specialty
- The bell-shaped staffing curve
- Staffing variation based on practice ownership
- The relationship between staffing and productivity
- The relationship between staffing and profitability
- Staffing in better-performing medical practices

STAFFING BY SPECIALTY

Medical practices staff at very different levels depending on their specialty. Exhibit 2.1 outlines the industry norms for total FTE support staff per FTE physician by practice specialty.

As demonstrated by these data, a practice specializing in family medicine typically has more staff than an anesthesiologist's or surgeon's practice. Family medicine physicians devote most of their time in the ambulatory care setting, whereas anesthesiologists work almost exclusively in a hospital or ambulatory surgery center and surgeons split their time between the office and the ambulatory surgery center or hospital, where they have a separate team to support their work. Thus, the appropriate volume and type of staffing will vary based on specialty.

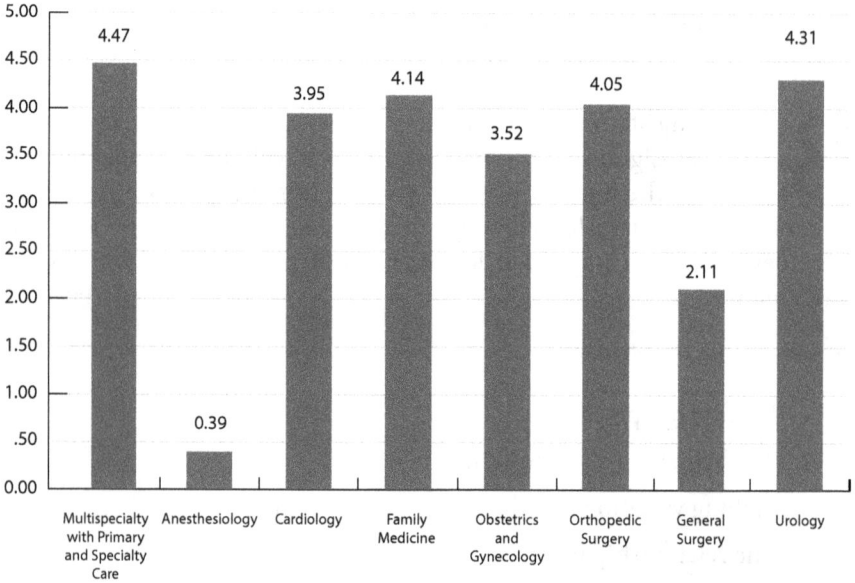

MGMA DataDive for Cost and Revenue 2017 Report Based on 2016 Data. Copyright 2017 MGMA. All
rights reserved. Reprinted with permission.

THE BELL-SHAPED STAFFING CURVE

When we standardize staffing levels by dividing the total support staff by the
number of FTE physicians and graph the staffing levels of all practices in a
specific specialty, we typically see a bell-shaped curve. That is, practices will
staff at very different levels, with the ends of the curve having a few practices
with substantially lower and higher staffing levels than most practices that
are in the middle, forming a curve that has a bell shape. For some, this is
counterintuitive, as it seems reasonable that staffing among practices of the
same specialty would have similar staffing patterns.

Practices of the same specialty will often offer different services. As an
example, an orthopedic practice may have its own imaging and hence have

a different staffing model than a peer orthopedic practice that does not offer this service in-house. As another example, a primary care practice that performs stress echo tests, DEXA scans and other procedures or one that has its own in-house laboratory will have a staffing model that differs from peer primary care practices that only offer office-based visits. Yet even when similar services are offered in two practices of the same specialty, one practice will often staff differently than its peer.

Importantly, a similar pattern exists in every specialty; the numbers and percentages reported in the graph will change by specialty but the graph maintains a bell shape.

STAFFING VARIATION BASED ON PRACTICE OWNERSHIP

The type of ownership of a medical practice also impacts staffing levels. Exhibits 2.2 and 2.3 display how physician-owned and hospital-owned multispecialty groups with primary and specialty care have different staffing patterns, yet have similar bell-shaped curves.

In Exhibit 2.2 we learn that the most frequent staffing model (representing 37% of practices reporting) for multispecialty practices that are physician-owned is 5.1 to 6.0 FTE staff per FTE physician. For hospital-employed multispecialty practices, the most frequent staffing model (representing 35% of practices reporting) is 3.1 to 4.0 FTE staff per FTE physician, as depicted in Exhibit 2.3.

In this case, the ownership of the practice — whether it is physician-owned or hospital-owned — impacts the staffing levels of the medical practice, with hospital-owned practices typically exhibiting lower staffing levels than their physician-owned counterparts.

Exhibit 2.2 Bell-Shaped Staffing Curve for Physician-Owned Multispecialty Groups with Primary and Specialty Care[2]

FTE Employees per FTE Physician for Physician-Owned
Multispecialty Groups with Primary and Specialty Care

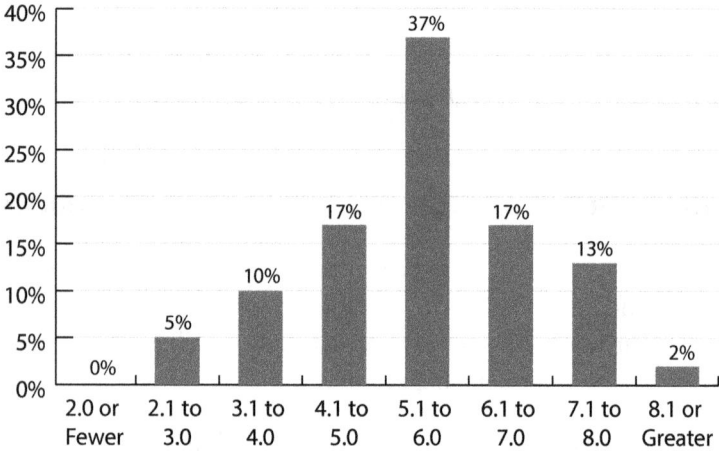

Exhibit 2.3 Bell-Shaped Staffing Curve for Hospital-Owned Multispecialty Groups with Primary and Specialty Care[3]

FTE Employees per FTE Physician for Hospital/IDS-Owned
Multispecialty Groups with Primary and Specialty Care

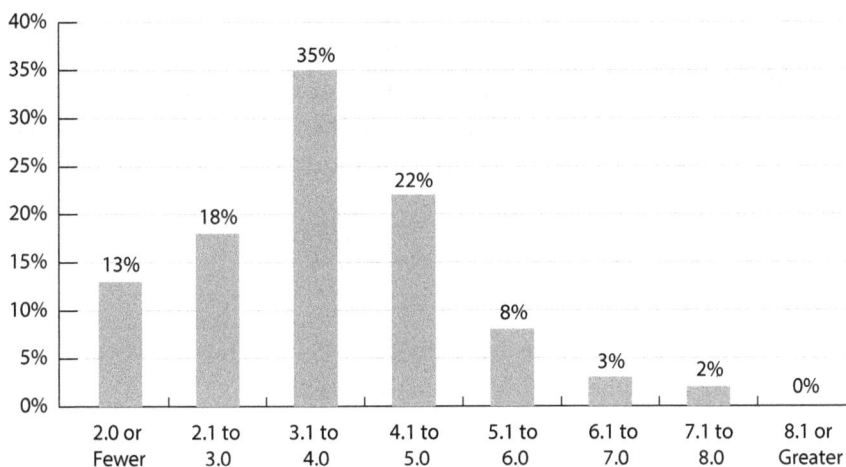

Range	Percentage
2.0 or Fewer	13%
2.1 to 3.0	18%
3.1 to 4.0	35%
4.1 to 5.0	22%
5.1 to 6.0	8%
6.1 to 7.0	3%
7.1 to 8.0	2%
8.1 or Greater	0%

The Relationship Between Staffing and Productivity

Many medical practices make the incorrect assumption that they should simply staff at industry norms. Often reflected by the median, this is the midpoint of a distribution where one half of the practices in the dataset report fewer staff and one half of the practices report more staff than this midpoint level. When medical practices revert to the median, they ignore the full story told by the data and disregard the relationships between data measures that further inform the optimal staffing for a medical practice.

When we combine different measures in a graph, we are able to see relationships between each criterion. In the case of staffing a medical practice, what we truly seek to learn is the level of staffing needed to optimize quality, profitability, practice efficiency, and customer experience. It is through the impact of one data element on another that we can begin to learn about optimal staffing levels in a medical practice.

Let's now examine the important relationship between staffing and productivity.

As shown in Exhibit 2.4, when work relative value unit (wRVU) production in multispecialty practices is separated into quartiles, distinct differences in staffing emerge between practices in the first quartile (those practices reporting the lowest productivity) and the fourth quartile (those practices reporting the greatest productivity).

Specifically,

- Practices that are the least productive have lower overall staffing levels than highly productive practices,
- Practices with the greatest productivity have approximately a quarter more clinical (nursing) support staff than practices with the lowest productivity,
- Practices with the greatest productivity have higher support staff costs (they have more staff and in some cases, also offer higher wage rates to their employees), and
- Importantly, the most productive practices also have the highest profitability defined as revenue minus operating costs. Revenue generation therefore exceeds the cost of the additional staff and increased general operating costs.

In sum, highly productive practices have more support staff and while they have higher support staff costs, the increase in revenue exceeds the higher expenses resulting in higher profitability for these practices. This demonstrates that their staff are well-deployed to the work. Thus, ensuring your practice is staffed at optimal levels has a direct impact on your practice's bottom line.

Exhibit 2.4 Staffing Levels, Revenue, and Cost by Work RVU Productivity for Physician-Owned Multispecialty Groups with Primary and Specialty Care[4]

Staffing Levels, Revenue, and Cost by Work RVU Productivity for Physician-Owned Multispecialty Groups with Primary and Specialty Care				
	Less than 6511 WRVUs per FTE Physician	6512 to 7307 WRVUs per FTE Physician	7308 to 8955 WRVUs per FTE Physician	8956 and greater WRVUs per FTE Physician
Staffing Levels				
Median total support staff per FTE physician	4.92	5.73	5.97	6.64
Median total business operations support staff per FTE physician	1.04	1.35	1.32	1.56
Median total front office support staff per FTE physician	1.46	1.41	1.33	1.42
Median total clinical (nursing) support staff per FTE physician	1.72	1.84	2.03	2.20
Median total ancillary support staff per FTE physician	0.64	0.92	0.82	1.15
Revenue and Expense				
Median total medical revenue per FTE physician	$918,834	$1,135,403	$1,190,076	$1,417,082
Median total support staff cost per FTE physician expense	$275,875	$348,680	$313,912	$342,154
Median total general operating cost per FTE physician	$272,627	$322,368	$406,324	$453,235
Median total medical revenue after operating cost per FTE physician	$330,056	$469,373	$418,710	$521,582

Medical Group Management Association 2017 DataDive Pro Cost and Revenue Quartile Report. Copyright 2017 MGMA. All rights reserved. Reprinted with permission.

To further examine the relationship between staffing and productivity, Exhibit 2.5 is a scatter plot that illustrates the relationship between staffing levels and procedure volumes (a measure of productivity in a medical practice). The number of FTE staff per FTE physician is reported on the x, or horizontal, axis and the number of procedures per FTE physician is reported on the y, or vertical, axis. A regression line is displayed allowing us to look at the path of the center of the data.

In this case, the regression line increases from left to right in the exhibit, suggesting that there is a positive relationship between the increase in staff and the increase in the number of procedures for a medical practice.

EXHIBIT 2.5 IMPACT OF TOTAL FTE SUPPORT STAFF PER FTE PHYSICIAN ON TOTAL PROCEDURES PER FTE PHYSICIAN IN MULTISPECIALTY GROUPS WITH PRIMARY AND SPECIALTY CARE[5]

IMPACT OF TOTAL FTE SUPPORT STAFF PER FTE PHYSICIAN ON TOTAL PROCEDURES PER FTE PHYSICIAN IN MULTISPECIALTY GROUPS WITH PRIMARY AND SPECIALTY CARE.

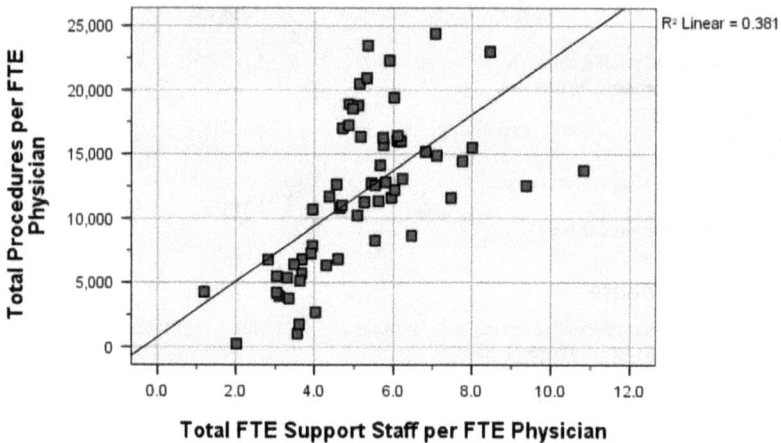

THE RELATIONSHIP BETWEEN STAFFING AND PROFITABILITY

In fact, not only does productivity increase with the number of FTE staff per FTE physician as demonstrated in Exhibits 2.4 and 2.5, but there is a positive relationship between the increase in staff and both total medical revenue and total operating costs, as depicted in Exhibits 2.6 and 2.7. (In both of these exhibits, the regression line increases from left to right as we saw in Exhibit 2.5.)

IMPACT OF TOTAL FTE SUPPORT STAFF PER FTE PHYSICIAN ON TOTAL MEDICAL REVENUE PER FTE PHYSICIAN IN MULTISPECIALTY GROUPS WITH PRIMARY AND SPECIALTY CARE.

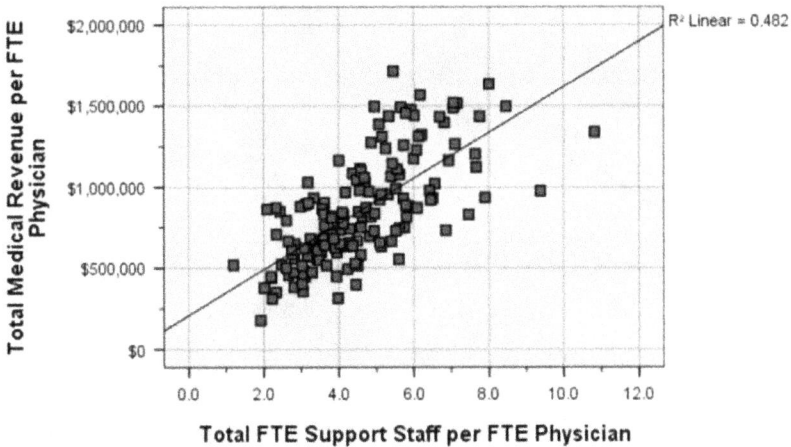

Custom analysis of the Medical Group Management Association 2016 Cost Survey database. Copyright 2017 MGMA. All rights reserved. Reprinted with permission.

EXHIBIT 2.7 IMPACT OF TOTAL FTE SUPPORT STAFF PER FTE
PHYSICIAN ON TOTAL OPERATING COST PER FTE PHYSICIAN
IN MULTISPECIALTY GROUPS WITH PRIMARY AND SPECIALTY
CARE[7]

IMPACT OF TOTAL FTE SUPPORT STAFF PER FTE PHYSICIAN ON TOTAL OPERATING COST PER FTE PHYSICIAN IN MULTISPECIALTY GROUPS WITH PRIMARY AND SPECIALTY CARE.

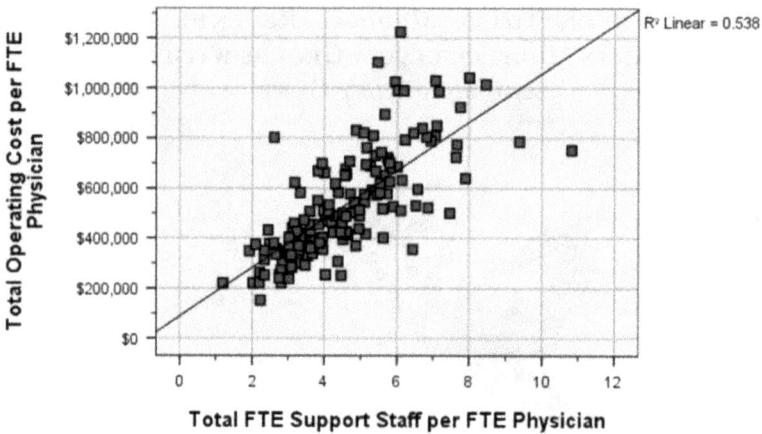

Exhibit 2.8 displays total medical revenue after total operating cost showing that there is a generally positive association between having an increased number of staff and practice profitability. This relationship between staffing levels and profitability is important. With staff costs typically representing more than 25% of the total medical revenue that is earned in a medical practice, the number, skill mix, and assignment of the staff are critical in terms of the overall profitability of a medical practice.

EXHIBIT 2.8 IMPACT OF TOTAL FTE SUPPORT STAFF PER
FTE PHYSICIAN ON TOTAL MEDICAL REVENUE AFTER TOTAL
OPERATING COST PER FTE PHYSICIAN IN MULTISPECIALTY
GROUPS WITH PRIMARY AND SPECIALTY CARE[8]

IMPACT OF TOTAL FTE SUPPORT STAFF PER FTE PHYSICIAN
ON TOTAL MEDICAL REVENUE AFTER OPERATING COST
PER FTE PHYSICIAN IN MULTISPECIALTY GROUPS WITH
PRIMARY AND SPECIALTY CARE.

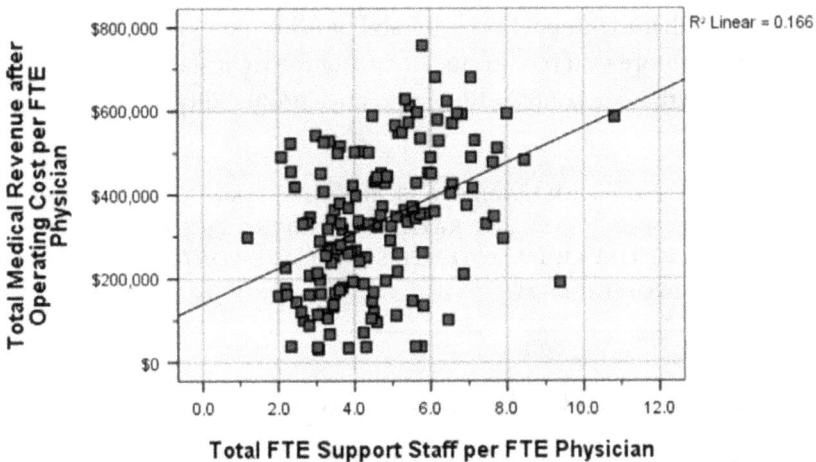

Thus, in general, total medical revenue, operating costs and total medical revenue after operating cost increase with the number of FTE staff per FTE physician. This suggests that there are significant benefits to investing in higher FTE staff levels.

However, it is important to further analyze the data to understand the connectivity between each of these elements. By analyzing staffing levels, revenue, expenses, and medical practice profitability together, we learn that:

- Typically, there is a strong positive relationship between more staff and productivity.

- The greater level of productivity has a proportional increase in total medical revenue.

- Since operating expenses also increase, the positive relationship between the number of staff and practice profitability is weak.

This suggests that the impact on profitability is not necessarily the result of simply having more staff but, rather, of having the right staff performing the right activities that are contributing to practice profitability.

> THE IMPACT ON PROFITABILITY IS NOT NECESSARILY THE RESULT OF HAVING MORE STAFF BUT RATHER OF HAVING THE RIGHT STAFF PERFORMING THE RIGHT ACTIVITIES THAT ARE CONTRIBUTING TO PRACTICE PROFITABILITY.

STAFFING IN BETTER-PERFORMING PRACTICES

We have conducted extensive studies of the data and the relationships between data elements in "better-performing" medical practices. For this discussion, the criteria for the selection of better-performing medical practices are financially based, as opposed to those that may have better quality or better patient care outcomes. Financial performance has been selected because:

- It is more objective than other measures when differentiating performance among medical practices.

- It can be easily measured.

- For purposes of staffing, the financial measures also get to the heart of the business-of-medicine concerns related to staffing strategies in a medical practice.

We have learned three key staffing insights from the experiences of better-performing medical practices:[9]

- *Insight 1:* Better-performing medical practices tend to have a higher quantity of staff. They have more staff on a per FTE physician basis than their practice counterparts.

- *Insight 2:* The cost of staff on a per FTE physician basis is also higher. This could be due to any number of factors: (1) they have more staff, (2) the staff are paid higher wage rates, and/or (3) they have a different skill mix of staff.

- *Insight 3:* Although these groups have more staff and a higher cost of staff on a per FTE physician basis, since revenue also increases, many of these medical practices have *lower* staff costs as a percentage of total medical revenue (the percentage of overhead devoted to staffing).

This finding is exciting! It means that better-performing practices are reaping the benefits of their higher staffing levels even if they have higher staff costs on a per FTE physician basis by having the staff devoted to the right activities, making a positive contribution to practice profitability.

These insights are summarized in Exhibit 2.9.

EXHIBIT 2.9 INSIGHTS FROM BETTER-PERFORMING PRACTICES

Insight 1: Employ more staff
Insight 2: Maintain a higher cost of staff on a per-FTE-physician basis
Insight 3: Have lower staff cost as a percentage of total medical revenue (lower staff overhead costs)

SUMMARY

What do these data lessons mean for a typical medical practice?

First, it is important to understand staffing at the specialty-specific level and how your practice may differ from its peers and require more or fewer staff as you situate your practice on the bell-shaped staffing curve.

Second, the important relationships between staffing and productivity and profitability necessitate critical attention to staffing, to include altering staffing models over time to align with changing productivity and performance of your medical practice.

Third, we can import lessons learned from better-performing medical practices; to appropriately staff a medical practice, you need the right staff performing the right work — no more, no less.

ENDNOTES

1 MGMA DataDive for Cost and Revenue 2017 Report Based on 2016 Data. Copyright 2017 MGMA. All rights reserved. Reprinted with permission.

2 Ibid.

3 Ibid.

4 Ibid.

5 Custom analysis of the Medical Group Management Association 2016 Cost Survey database. Copyright 2017 MGMA. All rights reserved. Custom Analysis by David N. Gans.

6 Ibid.

7 Ibid.

8 Ibid.

9 Better-performing medical practices have been isolated from the MGMA datasets due to their higher performance in the areas of (1) profitability and cost management; (2) productivity, capacity, and staffing; or (3) accounts receivable and collections.

PART 2

HOW TO IDENTIFY THE RIGHT NUMBER AND SKILL MIX OF STAFF

CHAPTER 3

STAFF
BENCHMARKING

Guest Co-author: David N. Gans

In Chapter 2, we share important insights regarding staffing data and the critical relationships between staffing and both productivity and performance. In this chapter, we utilize staffing data to conduct benchmarking analysis to identify areas of staffing opportunity. Staff benchmarking is one of two tools that we recommend to address the question, "Do I have the right staff in my medical practice?" The second tool, discussed in Chapter 4, is to compare the current productivity of your staff to expected staff productivity workload ranges.

In this chapter, we present:

- Staff benchmark data
- Benchmark limitations
- Basic approach to staff benchmarking

STAFF BENCHMARK DATA

Benchmarking permits a medical practice to compare its staffing levels and staffing skill mix to similar practices. This is an important step in the staffing process because it permits a medical practice to identify where its staffing model may be different or at variance with the benchmark data.

Let's look at the staff benchmark data that are available for us as we determine whether a medical practice has the "right staff."

Exhibit 3.1 outlines the staffing data that are included in MGMA's annual Cost and Revenue Survey. The staffing benchmark data are reported in the MGMA DataDive Cost and Revenue web-based reporting platform and in the printed MGMA Cost and Revenue Report.

Exhibit 3.1 Staffing Benchmarks[1]

Staff Category	Staff Function
Business operations staff	General administrative Patient accounting General accounting Managed care administrative Information technology Housekeeping, maintenance, security
Front office support staff	Medical receptionists Medical secretaries, transcribers Medical records Other administrative support
Clinical support staff	Registered nurses Licensed practical nurses Medical assistants, nurse aides
Ancillary support staff	Clinical laboratory Radiology and imaging Other medical support services

Source: Medical Group Management Association. Cost and Revenue Survey Report. Note: These are standard definitions used each year. Reprinted with permission.

In the left column of the exhibit, there are four main categories of staff that are reported in the benchmark data set:

1. **Business operations:** Business and administrative staff, to include general administrative services, revenue cycle, information technology and facilities support,

2. **Front office support:** Staff supporting communications, patient check-in, and patient check-out functions,

3. **Clinical support:** Nursing and medical assisting staff involved in the clinical services provided by the medical practice, and

4. **Ancillary support:** Staff performing clinical laboratory and imaging services, and other medical support services.

The right column of the exhibit expands each staff category into specific job functions. The benchmark data are provided at both levels in the survey instruments: job category and job function. For example, in the category of clinical support staff, the data are reported separately for each function: registered nurses (RNs), licensed practical nurses (LPNs), and medical assistants (MAs), and are also summarized in one category as total clinical support staff.

The following sections outline the four key staffing benchmarks that are used by medical practices to evaluate their staffing levels.[2]

BENCHMARK 1: FTE STAFF PER FTE PHYSICIAN

This benchmark reflects the number of full-time equivalent (FTE) staff in comparison with the number of FTE physicians in the medical practice. By full-time equivalent, we mean the number of staff and physicians that you consider in your medical practice to be full-time. Note that this definition varies among medical practices. For example, some medical practices consider a 35-hour workweek to be full-time, while others consider full-time as a 40-hour workweek. This definition is left up to each medical practice.

Calculation: The benchmark of FTE staff per FTE physician is reported as a ratio. For example, if the data report 5.00 FTE support staff and 25.00 FTE physicians, the ratio is calculated as 5 divided by 25, or 0.20 staff FTE per FTE physician. If your staff consistently incur overtime, be sure to include this in the benchmarking analysis. For example, if Nurse Betty reports 10 hours of overtime each week, that is an FTE equivalency of 0.25 FTE. Isolated overtime does not need to be incorporated into the benchmarks; however, routine overtime should be included to recognize the true staffing volume in a medical practice.

The benchmark FTE staff per FTE physician essentially represents a macro-level comparison between medical practices of the same specialty to provide early identification of potential opportunity to alter the staffing levels or staffing deployment model in a medical practice. Note that we are saying "potential opportunity," because we need to migrate to a more detailed analysis to determine whether there is true opportunity to change staffing patterns in a medical practice.

The data for FTE staff per FTE physician are reported at the specialty level.

In some specialties, the data can also be reported separately, depending on whether the medical practice is considered a physician-owned practice or whether it is owned by a hospital or integrated delivery system.

In Exhibit 3.2, we provide an example of the data available by specialty for the FTE staff per FTE physician benchmark. Note that this is an example only. The actual benchmark data that should be used are the most current benchmark survey instrument and the data set that most closely resembles your medical practice (for example, peer medical practices of the same specialty or peer medical practices of the same specialty and the same ownership type).

Benchmark 2: FTE Staff per FTE Provider

A variation of the FTE staff per FTE physician benchmark is to compare the ratio of FTE staff to the FTE of all providers, to include not only physicians, but also nonphysician providers. A medical practice that employs nonphysician providers, to include nurse practitioners or physician assistants, should analyze FTE staff on a per FTE provider basis in addition to FTE staff per FTE physician.

This benchmark is also available in the MGMA data set and is defined as FTE staff per FTE provider. By evaluating FTE staff per FTE provider, we recognize the staffing needs that are required to support all providers (physicians and nonphysician providers) in a medical practice.

Exhibit 3.2 FTE Staff per FTE Physician in Multispecialty Groups with Primary and Specialty Care[3]

FTE Staff per FTE Physician in Multispecialty Groups with Primary and Specialty Care	
General administrative	0.35
Patient accounting	0.50
General accounting	0.06
Managed care administrative	0.10
Information technology	0.14
Housekeeping, maintenance, security	0.08
Total business operations support staff	**1.06**
Medical receptionists	1.03
Medical secretaries, transcribers	0.05
Medical records	0.12
Other administrative support	0.10
Total front office support staff	**1.16**
Registered nurses	0.36
Licensed practical nurses	0.33
Medical assistants, nurse aides	0.90
Total clinical support staff	**1.73**
Clinical laboratory	0.28
Radiology and imaging	0.25
Other medical support services	0.20
Total ancillary support staff	**0.66**
Total support staff	**4.47**

Medical Group Management Association, DataDive for Cost and Revenue 2017 Report based on 2016 Data. © 2017 MGMA. All rights reserved. Reprinted with permission. Note: Totals will not sum; median data is reported.

Calculation: The benchmark of FTE staff per FTE provider is reported as a ratio. For example, if the data report 5.00 FTE support staff and 30.00 FTE providers (including physicians and nonphysician providers), the ratio is calculated as 5 divided by 30, or 0.17 staff FTE per FTE provider.

In addition to benchmarking the quantity of staff on a per FTE physician and per FTE provider basis, the skill mix of staff in a medical practice can be benchmarked. This is accomplished by viewing the benchmark at the functional level, which helps a medical practice determine whether it has the right type of staff devoted to key functions.

For example, for clinical support staff, we compare a medical practice's clinical support staff at the categorical level, which is the total clinical support, and at the functional level, which involves comparing the mix of registered nurses, licensed practical nurses, and medical assistants in the practice. In each of these instances, we deploy the benchmark that is published for FTE staff per FTE physician (or per FTE provider). The difference only relates to the level by which we evaluate staffing, that is, whether it is by staff category (the total of all staff in the category, such as total clinical support staff) or staff function (the specific work functions or skill mix of the staff, such as RN, LPN, and MA).

BENCHMARK 3: STAFF EXPENSE PER FTE PHYSICIAN

Benchmark data are also available for analyzing staffing costs in a medical practice. One key benchmark is staff expense per FTE physician. This helps determine whether the cost of staff is in line with peer practices.

Calculation: This benchmark is reported at a dollar level and is calculated as staff expense divided by FTE physicians in the practice. For example, if the cost of staff salary and benefits is $100,000 in a medical practice and there are 5.00 FTE physicians, the calculation would be $100,000 divided by 5, or $20,000 per FTE physician.

To determine whether your support staff cost is in line with comparable medical practices, first calculate your cost on a per-FTE-physician basis and then compare it using the benchmarking survey data. Data are also available for each staff category and staff function. An example of this type of benchmarking data is provided in Exhibit 3.3.

EXHIBIT 3.3 STAFF EXPENSE PER FTE PHYSICIAN IN MULTISPECIALTY GROUPS WITH PRIMARY AND SPECIALTY CARE[4]

Staff Expense per FTE Physician in Multispecialty Groups with Primary and Specialty Care	
General administrative	$28,453
Patient accounting	$18,844
General accounting	$3,642
Managed care administrative	$3,926
Information technology	$8,069
Housekeeping, maintenance, security	$3,171
Total business operations support staff	**$59,434**
Medical receptionists	$30,178
Medical secretaries, transcribers	$1,800
Medical records	$4,095
Other administrative support	$3,150
Total front office support staff	**$35,811**
Registered nurses	$19,542
Licensed practical nurses	$15,364
Medical assistants, nurse aides	$29,337
Total clinical support staff	**$68,543**
Clinical laboratory	$11,867
Radiology and imaging	$12,740
Other medical support services	$10,218
Total ancillary support staff	**$27,128**
Total support staff	**$239,180**

Medical Group Management Association, DataDive for Cost and Revenue 2017 Report based on 2016 Data. © 2017 MGMA. All rights reserved. Reprinted with permission. Note: Totals will not sum; median data is reported.

Benchmark 4: Staff Expense as a Percentage of Total Medical Revenue

In our earlier discussion regarding better-performing practices, we learned that staff expense as a percentage of total medical revenue (or staff overhead cost) is lower for many better-performing medical practices. To determine if the overhead that is attributed to staff in your medical practice is consistent with benchmark data, first calculate your staffing expenditures. Expense includes compensation and benefits. Then compare this expense to the total medical revenue generated in your medical practice.

This, too, can be carried out at the level of staff category and staff function. In this manner, you can determine whether the overhead costs associated with staff in your medical practice are higher or lower than in other medical practices and identify areas where you might have cost-saving opportunities related to staff.

Calculation: The benchmark is reported as a percentage. As an example, if your staffing expense is $100,000 and total medical revenue for the practice is $300,000, the ratio is calculated at 0.33. In this example, 33% of total medical revenue is devoted to pay for staffing.

Exhibit 3.4 presents an example of the benchmarking data that are available for staff expense as a percentage of total medical revenue.

Exhibit 3.4 Staff Expense as a Percent of Total Medical Revenue in Multispecialty Groups with Primary and Specialty Care[5]

Staff Expense as a Percent of Total Medical Revenue in Multispecialty Groups with Primary and Specialty Care	
General administrative	3.04%
Patient accounting	1.96%
General accounting	0.35%
Information technology	0.82%
Housekeeping, maintenance, security	0.28%
Total business operations support staff	**6.33%**
Medical receptionists	3.29%
Medical secretaries, transcribers	0.15%
Medical records	0.41%
Other administrative support	0.39%
Total front office support staff	**4.31%**
Registered nurses	2.45%
Licensed practical nurses	1.71%
Medical assistants, nurse aides	3.58%
Total clinical support staff	**7.24%**
Clinical laboratory	0.99%
Radiology and imaging	1.29%
Other medical support services	1.29%
Total ancillary support staff	**3.03%**
Total support staff	**28.18%**

Medical Group Management Association, DataDive for Cost and Revenue. 2017 Report based on 2016 Data. © 2017 MGMA. All rights reserved. Reprinted with permission. Note: Totals will not sum; example of median data is reported.

Additional Staff Benchmarks

In addition to these four benchmarks, which are commonly used to identify opportunity to improve your staffing model, there are others that also can be used.

These include FTE staff per output of work:

- FTE staff per total relative value unit (tRVU)
- FTE staff per work relative value unit (wRVU)
- FTE staff per patient
- FTE staff per procedure

There are also staff benchmarks based on FTE staff per input of work: specifically, FTE staff per square feet of the medical practice.

Definitions for each measure are provided in the following sections.

FTE STAFF PER tRVU OR PER wRVU

The staffing needs in a medical practice vary based on the work that is performed in the practice. Staff benchmark data are reported for the sum of total relative value units (tRVU) and work relative value units (wRVU), which are medical practice production outputs. Since a physician will produce thousands of tRVUs and wRVUs per year, the staffing metric is usually calculated on a per 10,000 tRVU or 10,000 wRVU basis.

The tRVU has been determined to be the best standard measurement of total production, as it accounts for practice expense, malpractice risk and physician work. The wRVU is a subset of the tRVU: it has been determined to be the best standard measurement of physician work. As the scale of units are tied to procedure codes, the relative value units reflect the type of service provided to the patient. It's important to note that the Centers for Medicare & Medicaid Services, which maintains the Resource-based Relative Value Scale (RBRVS), issues annual updates. A limited number of tRVUs and wRVUs are impacted each year. Therefore, there may be fluctuations in the denominator of the ratio that require attention particularly when reviewing current data with historical results.

Calculation: This benchmark is expressed as a ratio. First determine your total RVU and work RVU levels and divide each of these by 10,000 to arrive at the denominator for each ratio. Then calculate the ratio as follows: FTE staff divided by the 10,000 total RVUs or 10,000 work RVUs values.

FTE STAFF PER PATIENT OR PER PROCEDURE

Another benchmark based on production output is FTE staff per patient. Staff are a step-fixed cost to a medical practice. That is, at some point an increase in patient volume signals the need for additional staff to be hired over current levels for certain work functions. When performing comparisons with other practices, it's vital to be consistent in the definition of "patients." Per the MGMA definition, this is the total number of individual patients who received services during the 12-month reporting period of the survey instrument.

Calculation: The benchmark is expressed as a ratio and is calculated as follows: FTE staff divided by the number of patients. (Note that a similar calculation can be derived by using total procedures, as the MGMA surveys also report FTE staff per total procedures.)

FTE STAFF PER SQUARE FOOT

The larger the medical practice, the more staff that are needed. This benchmark recognizes an input to the practice — the square footage of the practice's facility. Simply walking throughout a medical practice consumes valuable staffing resources and time. In addition, a medical practice with multiple practice sites will have more staff than a medical practice with a single site, with a full complement of staff required to support the internal patient flow process at each practice location.

Calculation: Since a practice has thousands of square feet the benchmark is calculated in a similar manner as wRVUs and tRVUs. The total square footage is divided first by 10,000 and this value is divided into the number of FTE staff.

More sophisticated medical practices use these additional benchmarks to refine their analysis and often develop staffing targets based on these measures. For example, a medical practice site may decide to increase staffing levels only when a targeted FTE staff per wRVU is achieved.

BENCHMARKING COMPARISON OF MULTIPLE PRACTICE SITES

The benchmarks can also be used to analyze the differences in staffing strategies for multiple practice sites within an organization. An example of this benchmarking is reported in Exhibit 3.5. The fundamental question that needs to be asked is: "What are the reasons for the differences among the practice sites?" It may be that there are legitimate reasons for the differences in staffing related to the specialty, the type of work performed, and the work quantity. However, it also may be that the staffing deployment models have migrated over time, and there is now an opportunity to realign staffing with the work throughout the organization.

In Exhibit 3.5, practice site A has a one-to-one assignment of a registered nurse to each 1.00 FTE physician. At site B, there is a combination of each type of clinical support staff; however, this site has more licensed clinical staff (RNs and LPNs) than the benchmark. The last site (site C) has an overall greater number of clinical staff per FTE physician compared with the other two practice sites, and it is higher than the benchmark. This is an excellent starting point for the analysis of clinical support staff for each site. The next steps are to evaluate physician productivity and the type of work delegated to the staff at each site.

EXHIBIT 3.5 MULTISITE COMPARISON OF STAFFING LEVELS: FTE STAFF PER FTE PHYSICIAN[6]

Job Function	Site A	Site B	Site C	Benchmark
Registered nurse	1.00	0.50	0.50	0.35
Licensed practical nurse	0.00	0.50	0.50	0.40
Medical assistant	0.30	0.50	1.00	0.95
Total clinical support staff	**1.30**	**1.50**	**2.00**	**1.60**

Note: Benchmark column will not total; sample median data is reported.

Benchmark Limitations

Benchmarking analysis helps you determine where your medical practice may have staffing opportunity. However, these data should not be used as absolute targets or goals absent an understanding of the benchmark limitations.

Four examples are provided here that showcase the limitations to the benchmarks to consider when interpreting the data. The purpose of drawing your attention to the benchmark limitations is to ensure that once you have benchmarked the staffing levels in your medical practice, you can translate the data into usable information to implement and improve your staffing model.

Work Tasks

Though the benchmark data are reported at the level of the job function, such as receptionist or registered nurse, it is not possible from these data to identify the specific work tasks that have been delegated to the staff. For example, a medical practice with a streamlined patient scheduling system will have fewer staff than a medical practice with a cumbersome scheduling process. So, a medical practice that offers advanced access where patients simply phone in or log onto the portal and are slotted for a same-day appointment will typically have fewer staff than a medical practice that requires the schedulers to take messages and obtain approval from a member of the care team for the same-day appointment. The work is less streamlined and less efficient in this latter practice.

As another example, the front office staff of two medical practices may perform very different work. In one medical practice, the staff may be required to manage inbound telephone calls, schedule patients, retrieve records from referring providers, conduct insurance verification and benefits eligibility, receive patients upon arrival, confirm coverage upon check-in, collect time-of-service payments, and arrive patients. In another medical practice, the work of the check-in staff may be limited to receiving and arriving patients, as administrative tasks are performed during scheduling, or via a kiosk or tablet check-in process. These two medical practices will have very different staffing levels, with the former likely having more front office staff due to the additional work tasks. If these two practices have the same staffing complement, the second medical practice will likely have staff with significant capacity.

TECHNOLOGY

The benchmark data have not been segmented relative to the level of technology used in a medical practice. For example, if a medical practice has a portal through which patients request appointments, request prescription renewals, obtain test results, and pay their bills, typically, fewer staff are required to manage the inbound telephone calls when compared with a medical practice that does not offer patients electronic access. As this example illustrates, the deployment and adoption of technology dramatically affects staffing levels.

PRODUCTIVITY

Staff levels in a medical practice represent a step-fixed cost; that is, as the practice becomes more productive, at some point more staff are needed to manage the work volume. The number of staff varies depending on a) the workload of the medical practice, b) the type of work (task) being performed, c) the tools and technology provided to the staff, and d) the time available to the staff member to complete the task. For example, a determination of the appropriate number of staff to manage inbound telephone calls is dependent on the volume of inbound communications received, the tasks and tools involved, and the time the staff members have to conduct their tasks.

As productivity increases, current staff FTE levels may be insufficient to permit work of high quality and a medical practice may hire more staff. For example, if a task can be performed in 10 hours per week, and there is a part-time staff member available, the medical practice may hire an additional 0.25 FTE. A medical practice with high productivity will typically have more, not fewer, staff to assist with its work; however, it is difficult at the staff benchmarking level to discern the variability in work productivity related to a specific task.

NUMBER OF PRACTICE SITES

As medical practices set up additional sites throughout a community, they typically must hire more staff to work at the sites (this includes staff traveling from site to site, as travel time must be accounted). Thus, a medical practice that has developed a geographic distribution strategy throughout its community will likely have more staff than a practice that is based at only one site. Although the benchmark survey instruments report the number of practice sites in the entire data set for the specialty, the direct contribution of these additional sites to the benchmark data is not evident.

We typically observe that medical practices with multiple satellite sites have more staff than their peers and, in some cases, less productive staff. This is because a core cadre of staff is needed to staff the satellite site(s) regardless of patient volume levels, thereby negatively impacting the ability of the medical practice to take advantage of economies of scale.

Thus, there are significant limitations to the staff benchmark data. The staff benchmarks that were discussed earlier in this chapter do not permit the level of distinction related to work tasks delegated to staff, the use and leverage of technology, practice productivity, and number of practice sites. However, the staff benchmarks are effective in identifying areas of opportunity in staffing that require further analysis.

> THERE ARE LIMITATIONS TO THE BENCHMARK DATA. DESPITE THESE LIMITATIONS, BENCHMARK STAFF LEVELS AND COSTS TO PEER PRACTICES TO IDENTIFY OPPORTUNITIES FOR IMPROVEMENT.

BASIC APPROACH TO STAFF BENCHMARKING

The benchmarking process is simple and straightforward. First, identify the key work functions that you have asked your staff to perform. Then identify the hours typically needed by the staff to perform these functions each week to derive an FTE level that is devoted to each function.

For example, let's say you have Bob working the front office and medical assistant Sally retrieving and rooming patients, and they both work full-time (in this example, a 40-hour workweek) in the medical practice. Exhibit 3.6 reflects the hours per week and the FTE devoted to each of their work functions.

Exhibit 3.6 Basic Benchmarking Example

Name	Work Function	Hours Per Week	FTE
Bob	Medical receptionist	40	1.00
Sally	Medical assistant	40	1.00
Total		**80**	**2.00**

Of course, the staffing patterns in many medical practices tend to be a bit more complicated than this example. For example, at times Bob may be assigned to work in the business office to conduct patient collections and Sally may be assigned to manage scheduling calls. If this is the case, simply approximate the hours per week that each staff member devotes to specific work functions in the practice. As demonstrated in Exhibit 3.7, Bob and Sally now have new work functions and FTE designations, given their multitasking assignments, though their total FTE will remain the same at 1.00 FTE each and the total FTE staff for the practice (in this case, 2.00 FTE) remains unchanged.

Exhibit 3.7 Basic Multitasking Benchmarking Example

Name	Work Function	Hours Per Week	FTE
Bob	Check-in/out	30	0.75
	Patient Collections	10	0.25
Subtotal		*40*	*1.00*
Sally	Medical assistant	20	0.50
	Scheduling	20	0.50
Subtotal		*40*	*1.00*
Total		**80**	**2.00**

In the example in Exhibit 3.7, Bob typically devotes 30 hours per week or 0.75 FTE to patient check-in/check-out processes and 10 hours per week or 0.25 FTE to patient collections.

We then map these work functions to the MGMA survey definitions. The work function listed for each staff is the one that most closely matches the operational definitions provided in the benchmark survey instrument. Per the MGMA survey definitions patient check-in and patient check-out falls under the survey work function of "medical receptionist," while patient collections falls under the work function of "patient accounting." Bob would be categorized as 0.75 FTE medical receptionist and 0.25 FTE patient accounting.

On the other hand, Sally typically divides her time between medical assisting activities and scheduling, devoting about 20 hours each week to each of these functions. In her case, when her work functions are mapped to the MGMA survey definitions, she is now reclassified as 0.50 FTE medical assistant and 0.50 FTE medical receptionist, as scheduling is one of the tasks included in the survey operational definition for medical receptionists.

Once we have applied this process to each staff member in the medical practice, we have the baseline data from which to benchmark a host of indices related to the number, skill mix, and cost of your staff.

Continuing with our benchmark example, let's assume there are three physicians who work full-time in the medical practice in which Bob and Sally work. The FTE staff per FTE physician is calculated in Exhibit 3.8 and is reported as a ratio.

EXHIBIT 3.8 CALCULATING FTE STAFF FTE PER FTE PHYSICIAN

Key Work Functions	Staff FTE	FTE Staff per FTE Physician
Medical reception	1.25	0.42
Medical assistant	0.50	0.17
Patient accounting	0.25	0.08
Total	**2.00**	**0.67**

This ratio, FTE staff per FTE physician, is typically the first benchmarking analysis that is conducted to determine if there is staffing opportunity in a medical practice. Using the example in Exhibit 3.8, we compare the total staff level of 0.67 FTE staff per FTE physician with the benchmarks for total FTE staff per FTE physician for similar medical practices.

We then look at the specific categories of the staff and compare the subtotals at the categorical level with the benchmarks (for example, the category of total clinical support staff). Finally, we expand the categorical level to the work function level and use this to also compare staff levels (for example, registered nurses, licensed practical nurses, and medical assistants — the work functions that are added together to create the categorical level of total clinical support staff).

By benchmarking staff to both the categorical and functional staffing levels, we move beyond the overall number of FTE staff per FTE physician or per FTE provider to recognize the roles and skill mix of the staff. At each level, we take a "deeper dive" into identifying potential staffing opportunity in comparison to peer medical practices.

BENCHMARKING STAFF COSTS

Now that we have benchmarked the quantity of staff and the skill mix of staff in the medical practice, we turn to the cost of staff and the benchmarks that are available for this analysis. There are two key benchmarks available for staffing cost analysis: (1) staff cost per FTE physician and (2) staff cost as a percentage of total medical revenue. The term "cost" in the MGMA survey instruments includes salaries, bonuses, incentive payments, profit distributions, and employee voluntary salary deductions made to retirement plans. It does not include staff benefits which are separately reported in the survey under "staff benefits."

By benchmarking staff cost in a medical practice, you can determine if you are paying more or less for staff in comparison to the benchmarks (defined as staff cost per FTE physician). This may be a function of the cost of individual staff, for example, higher wages than comparable practices or it may be due to the number of staff hired by the practice.

Continuing with our basic benchmarking example, to benchmark staff cost per FTE physician, first identify the salary and other payments for each staff member and then assign that cost based on FTE to each of the staff member's work functions. This is reported in Exhibit 3.9.

Exhibit 3.9 Staff Cost per Work Function

Name	Salary and Other Payments	FTE per Work Function	Salary and Other Payments Per Work Function
Bob	$30,800	0.75 medical receptionist 0.25 patient accounting	$23,100 $ 7,700
Sally	$35,200	0.50 medical assistant 0.50 medical receptionist	$17,600 $17,600
Total	**$66,000**	**2.00 FTE**	**$66,000**

Then assign the cost on a per FTE physician basis. Assuming that three physicians work in this medical practice, divide the salary per work function by 3.00 FTE physicians. This is reported in Exhibit 3.10. As demonstrated by the data, overall staff cost per FTE physician is $22,000, with $13,567 assigned to medical reception, $5,867 to medical assistant and $2,567 to patient accounting functions. Once these data are computed for the medical practice, compare the data to available benchmarks to measure the staff cost per work function per FTE physician against peer practices.

Exhibit 3.10 Staff Cost per FTE Physician by Work Function

Work Function	Staff Cost	Staff Cost per FTE Physician
Medical reception	$40,700	$13,567
Medical assistant	$17,600	$5,867
Patient accounting	$7,700	$2,567
Total	**$66,000**	**$22,000**

Finally, compare the cost of staff as a percentage of total medical revenue to peer practices. Continuing with our example, let's suppose that the three physicians generate $500,000 in medical revenue. In this basic example, total staff cost as a percentage of total medical revenue is calculated as 13.2% ($66,000 divided by $500,000).

Once this is calculated, take a deeper dive into the data and compare staff cost as a percentage of total medical revenue at the staff category and work function levels to the benchmarks. This tells you whether the amount of overhead attributed to staff based on staff category and work function is higher or lower than similar medical practices.

Note that beyond staff cost you can also benchmark your staff wages with other practices. There are many benchmarking sources that are available for this comparison, to include the MGMA DataDive Management and Staff Compensation data set, Bureau of Labor Statistics (BLS), vendor healthcare salary surveys, and other wage reports. Offering a competitive market wage rate is an obvious requirement for effective staff recruitment and retention.

Beyond staff cost comparisons, you also can determine if the *total support staff costs* in your practice are in line with other medical practices. By total support staff cost we mean a combination of staff cost (to include salaries, bonuses, incentive payments, profit distributions, voluntary employee salary deductions to retirement plans), as well as employee benefit costs. By calculating this total support staff cost and dividing it by total medical revenue you can compare your support staff operating overhead with other medical practices.

The staff benchmarking process is an important step to determine if you have the right number of staff and the right skill mix of staff, as well as whether you are paying competitive wage rates and benefits. However, importantly, staff benchmarking does not relate to productivity of the staff. Thus, you may have the requisite volume of staff and the right skill mix of staff, but if they are not performing at expected productivity levels, your practice may have significant improvement opportunity related to staffing.

Summary

In this chapter, we share industry staff benchmarks that are available to medical practices. It is important to recognize that each medical practice is unique and different, necessitating careful attention to determining the appropriate data to utilize when performing staffing benchmarking analysis. The data are available by specialty, practice ownership type and practice size, for example, so the most relevant benchmark data need to be identified prior to conducting the analysis.

We also share the basic steps in benchmarking staff in a medical practice. These include benchmarking the quantity of staff, the skill mix of staff, and the cost of staff. By benchmarking the staff in your medical practice to peer practices, you learn areas of potential opportunity to improve your staffing levels and staffing deployment model.

It is important to identify the skill needs of staff involved in medical practice work functions with the goals of matching staff to the required work function and ensuring expected levels of productivity and performance. Because staff productivity related to assigned work tasks is not directly considered in the staffing benchmarking process, in the next chapter, we evaluate the productivity of staff and compare this to expected staff productivity ranges to determine if the staff are more, or less, productive than comparable practices. By utilizing both staff benchmarks and productivity measures, you have the data needed to answer the question, "Do I have the right number and skill mix of staff in my medical practice?"

Endnotes

1 Medical Group Management Association. Cost and Revenue Report. Note: These are standard definitions used each year. Reprinted with permission.

2 Benchmark data from MGMA are cited in this book. Please note that specialty and state societies may also have relevant data for benchmarking purposes.

3 MGMA DataDive for Cost and Revenue 2017 Report Based on 2016 Data. Copyright 2017 MGMA. All rights reserved. Reprinted with permission.

4 Ibid.

5 Ibid.

CHAPTER 4

STAFF PRODUCTIVITY

W e have now benchmarked the staffing levels and staff costs in the medical practice. Through the benchmarking process, we have identified potential areas of opportunity to improve the staffing model. These are the areas that receive the initial focus as we work to refine our staffing analysis by comparing the staff's current workload levels with expected productivity levels for each key medical practice function.

In this chapter, we describe:

- The importance of staffing for the work
- Expected staff productivity for key work functions
- Data limitations
- How to interpret staff workload range data
- Basic approach to staff productivity analysis
- How to use productivity data to determine staff resource needs
- How to use productivity data to prevent work bottlenecks
- How to use predictive analytics to evaluate staff productivity

STAFFING FOR THE WORK

Although benchmarks are important and one method for determining whether a medical practice is staffed correctly, as we discuss in Chapter 3, Staff Benchmarking, there are limitations to the benchmarks. The actual productivity and specific tasks that have been delegated to staff in a medical practice are not recognized in the benchmarking process.

Similarly, if two medical practices have the same number of staff, yet patient volume is dramatically different, there may also be staffing opportunity, as one of the practices may have more (or fewer) staff than needed to manage this patient volume. Ideally, we want to staff for the actual work that is performed in a medical practice. The use of expected staff workload ranges helps to analyze staffing levels by considering the type of work and productivity or quantity of work performed by the staff.

Expected Staff Productivity for Key Work Functions

Productivity expectations, defined by expected staff workload ranges, are available for each key step in the patient flow and business processes of a medical practice.[1] The expected staff workload ranges were derived by interacting with employees during their work and observing the approximate time the staff took to perform each of their key work functions. The workload ranges are based on a seven-hour productive day in the medical practice (with one hour allocated to breaks and other non-productive time).

> Productivity expectations vary depending on the type of work that has been delegated to the staff to perform.

There are different productivity expectations depending on the type of work that has been delegated to the staff to perform. As examples:

Patient Check-in: If a staff member assigned to work patient check-in is responsible for validating information, conducting insurance verification, and obtaining time-of-service payments, the expected volume of patients to be checked in is lower when compared with a staff member who is only tasked with receiving and arriving patients due to the use of self-check-in protocols for patients via their smart phones, or a tablet or kiosk available upon entry to the practice.

Inbound Communication: The type of inbound communication determines the time needed to respond to the requestor and the skill mix needed for the staff to manage the communication. A secure, electronic message about concerns related to an adverse reaction to a new medication, for example, typically takes longer than an inbound call that involves rescheduling an existing appointment to a new date and time.

Thus, the expected workload ranges are broad, taking this work variation into account. When utilizing staff workload range data, we recommend validating the ranges in this book: a) to determine if they are appropriate and consistent for your specific situation, and b) to identify whether to target productivity at the lower, middle, or higher end of the range for your practice. By comparing the current productivity of the staff to anticipated productivity via the use of staff workload ranges, we begin to understand the variation in staffing that may have been created due to the work volume and work processes of the medical practice.

Exhibits 4.1 through 4.4 report the expected staff workload ranges for each key step in the patient flow process:

- Communications, including telephone management, and scheduling (see Exhibit 4.1);

- Front office, including registration, check-in, check-out, and referral management (see Exhibit 4.2);

- Clinical support, including nurse triage (via telephone and portal), visit support, and panel management (see Exhibit 4.3); and

- Business office, including credit and refund management, insurance account follow-up, and patient account follow-up (see Exhibit 4.4).

EXHIBIT 4.1 PRODUCTIVITY EXPECTATIONS FOR COMMUNICATIONS[2]

Work Function	Per Day	Per Hour
Telephones with messaging	300–500	42–71
Telephones with routing (electronic system) only	1,000–1,200	142–171
Appointment scheduling with mini-registration	75–125	11–18
Appointment scheduling with full registration	50–75	7–11

Source: Woodcock, Elizabeth W. and Deborah Walker Keegan. 2018. Patient Access: Tools and Strategies for the Medical Practice, Englewood, CO, MGMA. Reprinted with permission.

EXHIBIT 4.2 PRODUCTIVITY EXPECTATIONS FOR FRONT OFFICE[3]

Work Function	Per Day	Per Hour
Pre-visit or on-site financial clearance	60–80	9–11
Patient check-in -With data verification only -With data verification and cashiering	100–130 75-100	14–19 11-14
Check-out -With scheduling and cashiering -With scheduling, cashiering, charge entry	70–90 60-80	10–13 9-11
Referrals (inbound or outbound)	70–90	10–13

Source: Walker Keegan, Deborah and Elizabeth W. Woodcock. 2106 The Physician Billing Process: Navigating Potholes on the Road to Getting Paid. Englewood, Colo.: Medical Group Management Association. Reprinted with permission.

EXHIBIT 4.3 PRODUCTIVITY EXPECTATIONS FOR CLINICAL SUPPORT[4]

Work Function	Per Day	Per Hour
Nurse triage/advice via telephone or via portal	65–85	8-12
Patient intake: Patient rooming, vital signs	Variable based on specific work that can be delegated; typically, 25 to 40 patients per day	N/A
Visit support: Nurse visit support, procedures, education	Variable based on specific work that can be delegated; typically, 25 to 40 patients per day	N/A
Panel management/ health and wellness coaching	Variable, based on type and breadth of services provided. See Chapter 9: Staffing for Value-Based Care for a detailed discussion	N/A

N/A = not applicable

Note: The expected staff workload range assumes full nurse triage and advice, not simply prescription renewals or responding to inquiries of a nonclinical nature, such as scheduling or information requests.

Source: Woodcock, Elizabeth W. and Deborah Walker Keegan. 2018. Patient Access: Tools and Strategies for the Medical Practice, Englewood, CO, MGMA. Reprinted with permission.

Exhibit 4.4 Productivity Expectations for the Business Office[5]

Work Function	Per Day	Per Hour
Credits researched and processed	60-80	9-11
Insurance follow-up and action	50-70	7-10
Patient follow-up and action	70-90	10-13

Source: Walker Keegan, Deborah and Elizabeth W. Woodcock. 2016. The Physician Billing Process: Navigating Potholes on the Road to Getting Paid. Englewood, Colo.: Medical Group Management Association. Reprinted with permission.

The "Potholes" book contains additional expected staff workload ranges related to billing; the above exhibit reports a subset of this data.

We use the data displayed in these exhibits in the following chapters as we "build" the optimal staffing model for key work functions in the medical practice.

Limitations of Staff Workload Ranges

There are two important limitations to using expected staff workload range data in determining a staffing strategy for a medical practice. First, the workload ranges only relate to the *quantity* of work, not the *quality* of work that is performed, to include accuracy and customer service. Staff are not robots, and day-to-day practice operations are not always routine; that is one reason we noted earlier that we consider a productive day to be seven hours, not the typical eight hours.

You may need to relax the expected workload ranges for your employees if quality is not at the anticipated level until you can assess the reason staff are not able to perform at these levels. We also recommend initial focus on the lower end of the productivity ranges for newly trained staff, or staff who have been asked to learn new skills, with a defined timeframe for their learning curve (for example, three to six months depending on assigned work function and current level of skill, knowledge, and abilities).

> STAFF ARE NOT ROBOTS, AND DAY-TO-DAY PRACTICE OPERATIONS
> ARE NOT ALWAYS ROUTINE. EXPECTATIONS REGARDING STAFF
> PRODUCTIVITY MUST ALSO ACCOUNT FOR WORK QUALITY AND
> LEARNING CURVES FOR NEW EMPLOYEES AND STAFF ASSIGNED
> NEWLY DELEGATED WORK.

Secondly, the ability to perform within these workload ranges may vary due to internal, practice-specific factors such as your facility, technology, and the specific processes that the staff have been tasked to perform. Some medical practices have adopted streamlined processes, while others have encumbered processes with more steps, work hand-offs, and other complexities. It is important to verify that the expected staff workload range — and the position within that range that you adopt — is consistent with the productivity expectations reasonable for your own medical practice.

HOW TO INTERPRET STAFF WORKLOAD RANGE DATA

If there is a gap between the quantity of work that is performed by your staff and the expected workload range, ask the question: "why?"

If staff are performing at lower productivity levels than expected, potential reasons could include:

- The staff are highly multitasked, with limited time devoted to the task, and/or
- Work processes are highly encumbered, thereby creating inefficiencies.

You may have an opportunity to provide additional education to your staff, learn from others, and import best practices, or you may have an opportunity to innovate your work processes via technology.

In contrast, if your staff are performing at higher productivity levels than anticipated, potential reasons could include:

- Management, training and/or culture promotes productivity,
- Operational innovations permit staff to outperform other practices, and/or
- The work quality may not be at the projected level.

Your practice could be a "best" practice or it could suggest the need to evaluate work quality to ensure it is optimized.

By conducting a productivity gap analysis — comparing the workload levels currently handled by your staff to the expected staff workload ranges — important questions are raised that should be considered when evaluating your staffing levels. For example:

- Why are staff performing at levels that vary from the expected range?
- Is our work process streamlined or encumbered? Is there a work redesign opportunity?
- Is there a better way or better time to perform this work function, for example by pulling work into the practice versus conducting it at the back end?
- Can technology be leveraged to improve this work process?
- What best practices can be learned from others? Have other medical practices adopted a more innovative staffing strategy?
- Is there opportunity to improve performance, outcomes and/ or patient experience?

> BY CONDUCTING A PRODUCTIVITY GAP ANALYSIS YOU ARE IN A BETTER POSITION TO DETERMINE WHETHER YOU HAVE THE RIGHT NUMBER OF STAFF DEVOTED TO A SPECIFIC WORK FUNCTION.

BASIC APPROACH TO STAFF PRODUCTIVITY ANALYSIS

Building a staffing model utilizing staff productivity analysis involves the following five steps.

1. Determine the Unit of Work

First, ascertain the unit of work for a defined job function. For example, in the case of a staff member assigned as a telephone operator, the unit of work is the inbound telephone call. In contrast, in the case of a staff member assigned to support in-office flow, the unit of work is the arrived patient visit.

2. Capture Data

Next, capture current data related to work volume. For example, in the case of the telephone operator, capture inbound telephone call volume by day of week and time of day and reason for call.

3. Evaluate Expected Staff Workload Ranges

Review the expected staff workload range for the work function under analysis. Ensure that the expected range is generally consistent with your medical practice's work productivity by measuring the duration of time it takes to complete the task so you can confirm (or adjust) the range. For example, for telephone operators, measure the average handle time of a telephone call; for medical assistants, determine the average time to room both new and established patients and perform clinical intake while complying with expected protocols for these tasks. Then compare these data with the expected range to determine congruence. If the expected workload range differs from your practice's actual work levels, modify the range for your medical practice in the near-term while you learn why your practice may be different.

4. Calculate Required Staff FTE

Apply the expected staff workload to your current work volume and calculate the required staff FTE necessary for the work volume.

5. Perform a Gap Analysis

In step 5, compare the calculated staff FTE with the current staff FTE you have allocated to the work to identify opportunity.

CASE STUDY

Let's proceed through these steps to evaluate staff productivity by using an example related to patient check-in.

1. Determine the Unit of Work

Establish the unit of work for patient check in, which equals the number of patients who arrive for their visit and are checked in each day.

2. Capture Data

Capture your practice's arrived patient visit volume for a representative week, by day. Exhibit 4.5 reflects the arrived patient volume by day of the week for our sample medical practice. Note that further refinements can be made with data captured at the level of half-day session and/or by time of day.

EXHIBIT 4.5 ARRIVED PATIENT VOLUME BY DAY OF THE WEEK

Day of Week	Mon	Tue	Wed	Thu	Fri
Arrived Patient Volume	200	150	100	75	35

3. Evaluate Expected Staff Workload Ranges

In most medical practices, one staff member devoted to patient check-in can check in 100 to 130 patients per day if the work involves receiving the patient and verifying information with the patient (as outlined in Exhibit 4.2). The staff workload ranges are based on a seven-hour productive day. This means that, on average, patient check-in takes 3.2 to 4.2 minutes per patient.

To effectively use the expected workload range in your medical practice, first determine if the time to perform that work function is consistent with your medical practice's experience. Do this by evaluating the average time it takes for a staff member to conduct this work in your medical practice. Ask the staff to record the times for patient check-in by patient for a one-week period or sit with the staff and observe the average time it takes them to complete check-in processes. Then verify the staff workload range. In this example, is the 3.2 to 4.2 minutes per patient time consistent with your practice and its work processes? If not, adjust the range.

For this example, let's assume that the expected workload range of 100 to 130 patients per day is consistent with that observed at the medical practice.

Let's further agree that we want to take a conservative approach and use 100 patients per day (or the lower end of the workload range) to analyze the quantity of work conducted by the current staff.

4. Calculate Required Staff FTE

Calculate the staff FTE levels required for the current work volume by dividing the arrived patient volume by the expected workload level – in this example, 100. For example, on Monday, the arrived patient volume is 200 patients. Divide that by 100 to learn that 2.00 FTE are required to manage this volume of work. Proceed in a similar fashion for each day of the week.

Exhibit 4.6 outlines these calculations for each day of the week for our sample practice.

EXHIBIT 4.6 REQUIRED STAFF FTE CALCULATION

Day of Week	Mon	Tue	Wed	Thu	Fri
Arrived Patient Volume	200	150	100	75	35
Required Staff FTE	2.00	1.50	1.00	0.75	0.35

5. Perform a Gap Analysis

After calculating the required staff FTE for the work volume, report your current staff FTE assigned to the work. In our sample medical practice, let's assume there are 2.00 FTE assigned to patient check-in each day of the week. The final step is to calculate the gap, which is defined as the estimated requirement for staff FTE less the current staff FTE.

Exhibit 4.7 reflects these calculations. As demonstrated by these data, our sample medical practice has an appropriate number of staff assigned to the work on Monday – the arrived patient volume requires 2.00 staff FTE and the practice has assigned 2.00 staff FTE to the work. Throughout the rest of the week, however, there is increasing capacity for the staff assigned to this work function, given the decline in patient volume each day of the week. On

Friday, for example, only 0.35 staff FTE are required for patient check-in, yet the practice has assigned 2.00 FTE to this work function, suggesting it is overstaffed by 1.65 FTE.

This exhibit features a phenomenon commonly found in medical practices, in which the staffing level is assigned based on the highest work volume of the week. While the staff FTE levels remain at this peak, the actual work volume diminishes throughout the week. The solution is not necessarily to lay off staff members every Thursday and Friday. Instead, there are opportunities to either level load provider schedules and address the consistency of patient volume to make better use of existing staff or to identify more flexible staffing strategies for the medical practice.

EXHIBIT 4.7 STAFF FTE GAP ANALYSIS

Day of Week	Mon	Tue	Wed	Thu	Fri
Arrived Patient Volume	200	150	100	75	35
Required Staff FTE	2.00	1.50	1.00	0.75	0.35
Current Staff FTE	2.00	2.00	2.00	2.00	2.00
Staff FTE Gap	0.00	0.50	1.00	1.25	1.65

We utilize the above 5-step approach in each of the following chapters as we build the optimal staffing model for key work functions of the medical practice.

HOW TO USE PRODUCTIVITY DATA TO IDENTIFY STAFF RESOURCE NEEDS

The expected staff workload ranges can also be used to identify the number of staff required to perform a certain project, function, or task. For example, a medical practice may decide to focus the telephones in a central call center. By utilizing the expected staff workload ranges, we can begin to identify the number of staff required to meet patient telephone demand.

As an example, let's assume that the medical practice receives 1,500 inbound telephone calls per day, with one third of the calls involving patient scheduling, one third requiring messages to be taken, and one third relating to clinical issues. Let's also assume that the medical practice wants to include nurse triage staff on the telephones to manage the clinical calls. In this scenario, we analyze the data and employ the expected staff workload ranges to identify the number of staff required for the volume and type of work, as demonstrated in Exhibit 4.8.

The data show that this sample medical practice will generally need to staff its new call center with 7.00 FTE telephone schedulers/message staff and 7.50 FTE nurse triage staff (assuming the midpoint of the calculated ranges). As we describe in Chapter 5, Staffing Communications, we recommend a further refinement of the data to identify the actual staff needed by day of week, session per day, and time of day, as well as to account for staff absences. However, this example demonstrates the valuable use of expected staff workload ranges to identify staffing levels required to carry out specific work functions.

Exhibit 4.8 Using Expected Productivity Data to Identify Staff FTE Requirements

Call Type	Call Volume 1,500 Inbound Calls	Expected Workload Range, Calls per Day	Number of Staff FTE Required
Appointment scheduling with mini-registration	500 calls	75–125	4.00–6.67
Message-taking	500 calls	300–500	1.00–1.67
Total Scheduling/ Message Staff			**5.00–8.34**
Nurse triage	500 calls	65–85	6.67–8.33
Total Nurse Triage Staff			**6.67–8.33**

Source: Expected workload range data are derived from Exhibit 4.1, Expected Staff Workload Ranges for Communications and Exhibit 4.3, Expected Staff Workload Ranges for Clinical Support.

How to Use Productivity Data to Prevent Work Bottlenecks

Expected staff workload levels also help to diagnose staffing challenges in a medical practice. Let's say, for example, that a staff member devoted full-time to patient check-in can be expected to check in 100 patients per day. Based on a seven-hour productive day, this translates to 14 patients per hour, or 4 minutes and 20 seconds for each patient. It is Monday morning in the medical practice, and at 8:30 a.m., 20 patients present at the same time to be checked in by this one staff member. What do we already know about the consequences of this staffing strategy of this medical practice? Not only will patients be queued for long periods of time, but there will also be a significant delay in rooming patients.

A static staffing model — staffing at the same level throughout the day regardless of patient volume — fails to account for the actual work that physically can be done by a single staff member within a specified time. This concept of creating variable staffing deployment consistent with the work is one of the themes of this book — staff for the work — and is further discussed in Chapter 11, Teleworking and Flexible Staffing.

How to Use Predictive Analytics to Evaluate Staff Productivity

Another useful approach to identify staff resource needs is to use predictive analytics to examine your current staffing model in relation to your practice's productivity (for example, as measured by encounters or wRVUs) to determine if staff are working at consistent levels.

In Exhibit 4.9, we share an example of this type of analysis. In this example, the medical practice experiences fluctuating work levels throughout the week, as demonstrated by the variable encounter volume reported by day of week. The practice has intuitively staffed at variable levels throughout the week to attempt to match staffing to the work. In this example, the practice has 3.00 FTE receptionists working on Monday and Tuesday, 2.00 FTE receptionists working on Wednesday and Thursday and 1.50 FTE receptionists working on Friday.

To determine if this staffing model is the correct model, ensuring each staff member works at the same level of productivity, we calculate the current staff FTE per encounter. As depicted in Exhibit 4.9, the staff FTE per encounter ranges from 0.022 to 0.030, suggesting that on certain days of the week the staff are less productive than others.

EXHIBIT 4.9. CURRENT STATE: STAFF FTE PER ENCOUNTER

Current State	Mon	Tue	Wed	Thu	Fri
Receptionist	3.00	3.00	2.00	2.00	1.50
Encounters	100	125	90	75	50
Staff FTE Per Encounter	0.030	0.024	0.022	0.027	0.030

We then apply predictive analytics to determine the staff FTE level needed to ensure a consistent staff productivity level. Let's assume that the productivity level of 0.030 staff FTE per encounter is the goal for this practice. As demonstrated in Exhibit 4.10, an increase in staff FTE working Tuesday, Wednesday and Thursday will enable the staff to work at consistent production levels on a per-encounter basis throughout the week.

EXHIBIT 4.10 REDESIGNED STAFFING MODEL: STAFF FTE PER ENCOUNTER

REDESIGN	Mon	Tue	Wed	Thu	Fri
Encounters	100	125	90	75	50
Required Staff FTE at 0.030/ Encounter	3.00	3.75	2.70	2.25	1.50
Current Staff FTE	3.00	3.00	2.00	2.00	1.50
Staff FTE Gap	0.00	+0.75	+0.70	+0.25	0.00

This is another example of 'staffing for the work', ensuring the staff perform a similar work volume.

SUMMARY

As we discuss in this chapter, it is important to not only benchmark staffing levels to survey instruments, but also to evaluate the current productivity of the staff and compare it with expected workload ranges. Through these two approaches — staff benchmarking and staff productivity comparison — you can identify opportunity related to staffing volumes and skill mix of staff. Armed with these data, you can then answer the question, "Do I have the right number and skill mix of staff?" and identify whether there is staffing opportunity in your medical practice.

In the chapters that follow, we build the optimal staffing models for each key function in the medical practice, including staffing for communications, front office, the encounter, business office, and value-based care. We also share innovative work redesign strategies to align with new technologies, new patient access channels, new value-based services, and new patient engagement strategies — each of which requires a change to the staffing model of a medical practice. It is critical to make sure that staff are performing the right activities if we seek to optimize our care team.

ENDNOTES

1 For more information on staff workload ranges, see: Woodcock, Elizabeth W. 2014. Mastering Patient Flow, 4th Edition, Englewood, Colo.: Medical Group Management Association.

Walker Keegan, Deborah and Elizabeth W. Woodcock. 2016. The Physician Billing Process: Navigating Potholes on the Road to Getting Paid. Englewood, Colo.: Medical Group Management Association.

Woodcock, Elizabeth W. and Deborah Walker Keegan. 2018. Patient Access: Tools and Strategies for the Medical Practice, Englewood, Colo.: Medical Group Management Association.

2 Woodcock, Elizabeth W. and Deborah Walker Keegan. 2018. Patient Access: Tools and Strategies for the Medical Practice, Englewood, Colo.: Medical Group Management Association. Reprinted with permission.

3 Walker Keegan, Deborah and Elizabeth W. Woodcock. 2016 The Physician Billing Process: Navigating Potholes on the Road to Getting Paid. Englewood, Colo.: Medical Group Management Association. Reprinted with permission.

4 Woodcock, Elizabeth W. and Deborah Walker Keegan. 2018. Patient Access: Tools and Strategies for the Medical Practice, Englewood, Colo.: Medical Group Management Association. Reprinted with permission.

5 Walker Keegan, Deborah and Elizabeth W. Woodcock. 2016. The Physician Billing Process: Navigating Potholes on the Road to Getting Paid. Englewood, Colo.: Medical Group Management Association. Reprinted with permission.

Part 3

How to Staff Key Patient Flow and Business Processes

CHAPTER 5

STAFFING
COMMUNICATIONS

In this chapter, we discuss how to optimally staff your inbound communications. In addition to the telephone, today's medical practice receives communications via secure, electronic messaging and the portal, requiring an effective staffing model for each of these communications channels and technologies. Unfortunately, in some medical practices, the communications management process is broken; the telephone rings off the hook or worse, goes to voicemail.

In this chapter, we:

- Discuss the importance of managing inbound communications
- Describe the traditional communications process
- Provide performance expectations for communications
- Build the communications staffing model
- Share innovative strategies for communications
- Provide key questions to address to staff for communications

IMPORTANCE OF COMMUNICATIONS MANAGEMENT

The staffing model deployed to manage inbound communications impacts the financial viability of a medical practice. Via the telephone and/or portal, we typically learn the patient's demographic and insurance information to permit us to bill for rendered services, obtain required referrals, and inform the patient regarding financial obligations.

Furthermore, optimal communications with patients is critical to patient health, safety and engagement. The telephone and/or portal are a pathway by which patients access appointments, learn of test results, seek (and receive) medical advice, request referrals and prescription renewals, and other similar tasks.

TRADITIONAL COMMUNICATIONS PROCESS

Although many medical practices are expanding their use of portals, secure messaging, and other electronic access methods, the telephone is still the technology typically used by patients, referring physicians, hospitals, nursing homes, pharmacies, and other stakeholders to contact the medical practice.

The traditional process for communications management is depicted in Exhibit 5.1. In this process, a medical practice uses an automated attendant to initially receive inbound telephone calls, with the caller selecting from a menu of options. For example, patients select 1 to schedule an appointment, 2 to talk to a nurse, and so forth. In some practices, the automated attendant is a staff member in the role of a telephone operator, manually distributing telephone calls after inquiring about the caller's needs.

As appropriate, telephone calls are managed by telephone operators/ schedulers who schedule the patient for a visit, transfer the call to an appropriate party, or take a message. Many messages relate to clinical issues, and these calls are either transferred to the clinical support staff or messages are transmitted to the nurse for resolution.

EXHIBIT 5.1 TRADITIONAL COMMUNICATIONS MANAGEMENT PROCESS

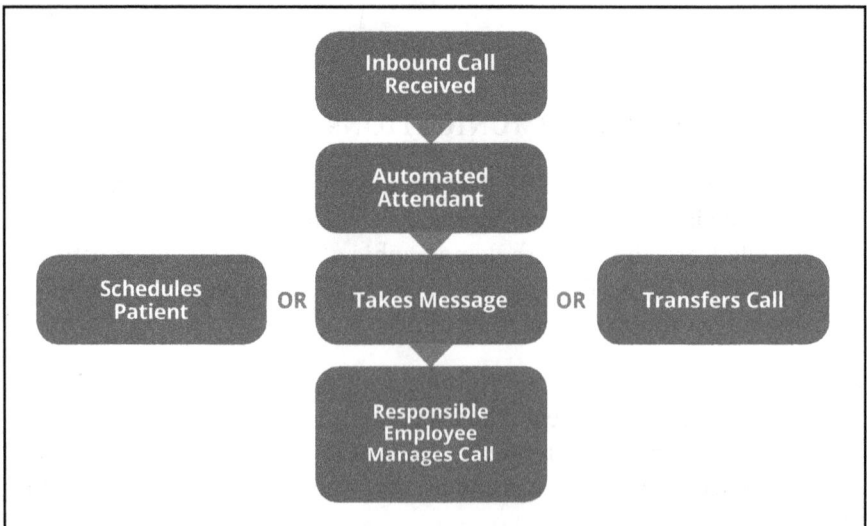

This traditional communications management process is costly and encumbered. We often hear complaints by patients, physicians, and staff alike. Some of the common complaints are listed in Exhibit 5.2.

EXHIBIT 5.2 COMMON COMPLAINTS REGARDING COMMUNICATIONS MANAGEMENT

Area	Performance Challenges
People	Inconsistent skill set Poor customer service Inconsistent information provided to patient Inaccurate scheduling
Messages	Insufficient message detail Inconsistent scripting with patient Incomplete reason for visit Unrealistic turnaround times provided to patients
Work processes	Long wait time on-hold Delays in returning calls to patients Telephone tag with patient for call-back Each call touched more than once

THE TRADITIONAL COMMUNICATIONS MANAGEMENT PROCESS FOR A MEDICAL PRACTICE IS COSTLY AND ENCUMBERED.

These complaints can be resolved with appropriate staffing strategies, including:

- The correct number of staff assigned to manage communications,
- The correct skill mix of staff assigned to communications,

- Performance expectations regarding care and service,
- Performance expectations regarding response turnaround time,
- Consistent, standard work processes, and
- Staff education and scripting.

PERFORMANCE EXPECTATIONS FOR COMMUNICATIONS MANAGEMENT

Make it easy for patients to reach you! Institute performance expectations for communications management, measure your staff's ability to achieve these standards, and create specific targets and goals for improvement, such as the following:

- Call abandonment rate: 3 percent or less
- Service level: 80 percent of calls answered within 30 seconds
- On-hold time: 30 seconds or less

Exhibit 5.3 outlines common expectations regarding communications management to get you started.

Exhibit 5.3 Performance Expectations for Communications Management[1]

Measurement	Standard
Abandonment rate	3 percent or less
Availability	85 percent or more, based on workday unless excused for training or other duties
Average handle time	Set in accordance with practice protocols; monitored by management with focus on after-call employee efficiency
Average speed to answer	24 seconds or less (maximum of four rings, if manually calculated)
Callback rate	Clinical: Within 30 minutes of initial call. All others: All calls acknowledged within three hours of receipt, regardless of ability to fully answer the request. Answer by end of day, unless extenuating circumstances. 100 percent of callbacks made, and performed within the established time frames.
Duration of call	Set in accordance with practice protocols; monitored by management but not a component of employee performance
Hours of operation	30 minutes before office hours begin until 5 p.m. Open continuously through the lunch period.
Message quality	100 percent
On-hold time	30 seconds or less
Script compliance rate	100 percent
Service	100 percent professionalism, courtesy, compassion, and empathy; use of service recovery
Service level	80 percent within 30 seconds
Staff occupancy	80 percent or more, but depends on size of operation and expected performance quality
Trunk blockage	0 percent

Woodcock, Elizabeth W. and Deborah Walker Keegan, 2018. Patient Access: Tools and Strategies for the Medical Practice, MGMA. Reprinted with permission.

Beyond these performance expectations, capture and evaluate data regarding the success of your practice's communications management process. Exhibit 5.4 lists the type of data that are routinely available to assess the appropriateness of a medical practice's staffing model devoted to the volume of calls and communications management performance.

EXHIBIT 5.4 DATA TO ASSESS COMMUNICATIONS STAFFING[2]

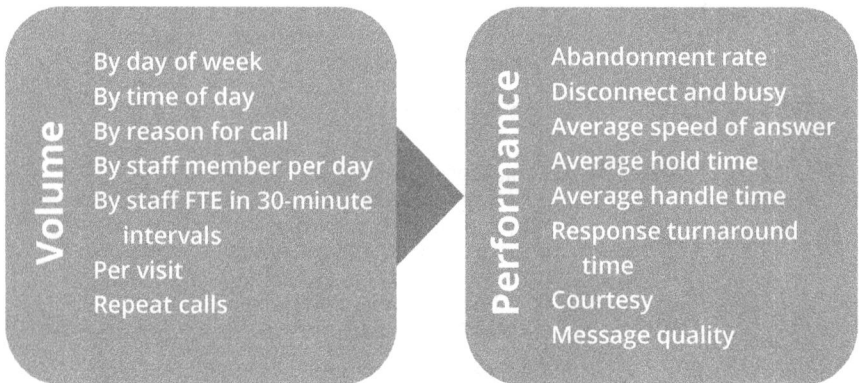

Volume	Performance
By day of week	Abandonment rate
By time of day	Disconnect and busy
By reason for call	Average speed of answer
By staff member per day	Average hold time
By staff FTE in 30-minute intervals	Average handle time
Per visit	Response turnaround time
Repeat calls	Courtesy
	Message quality

Woodcock, Elizabeth W. and Deborah Walker Keegan, 2018. Patient Access: Tools and Strategies for the Medical Practice, MGMA. Reprinted with permission.

Some of these measures are used to build the staffing model for communications management in a medical practice (discussed in the section below), to include inbound telephone volume by day of week, time of day and reason for call. Other measures help refine the staffing strategy for communications management once it is adopted. For example, the volume of calls managed within 30 minutes by each staff member helps identify potential performance gaps among staff. Staff may be spending too long on the telephone attempting to manage patients' inquiries because the staff need further education and training to handle them. Alternatively, some staff may be cutting the call short and are not able to gauge patients' needs to assist them and/or to take a complete and accurate message.

BUILDING THE STAFFING MODEL FOR COMMUNICATIONS

Follow these steps to build an optimal staffing deployment model for communications management. Be sure to construct a staffing deployment model specific to each of your inbound technologies. These include telephones, secure messaging, and portal communications. In this chapter, we demonstrate how to build an optimal staffing model to manage inbound telephone communications. A similar approach should be taken for each communication channel.

STAFF BENCHMARKING ANALYSIS

First, follow the steps outlined in Chapter 3, Staff Benchmarking to compare your staff FTEs and staff costs for telephone management to the benchmark.

Operational definitions in the MGMA survey instruments describe the type of staff included in each of the job categories and job functions for which benchmark data are reported. The work function of *medical receptionist* (reported under the staffing category of front office support staff) includes telephone operators and schedulers. For calls taken by clinical support staff, use the *registered nurse (RN), licensed practical nurse (LPN), or medical assistant (MA)* work functions (reported under the staffing category clinical support staff), depending on the licensure of staff involved in telephone management. Allocate the time expended by the RN, LPN, or MA respectively, for calls taken by clinical support staff.

The staff benchmarking data may alert you to outlier areas in your medical practice — where your practice differs from the benchmark. Staff benchmarking is the first step in determining areas of staffing opportunity.

STAFF PRODUCTIVITY ANALYSIS

After you have benchmarked your staff, follow the steps in Chapter 4, Staff Productivity, and outlined below, to analyze staff productivity and compare it to expected workload ranges. This assessment helps to identify the appropriate staffing FTE levels and staffing skill mix required to manage the volume and type of call.

1. Determine the Unit of Work

Recognize the unit of work for telephone staff, which is the volume of inbound telephone calls by call type that are managed by the staff.

2. Capture Data

Calculate the volume of inbound calls by day of week and time of day. To obtain inbound telephone call volume, determine whether your telephone system can provide this information. If not, simply ask the staff to collect these data for a one-week period. The goal is to obtain a representative sample of data.

Graph this information to learn more about the data. Exhibit 5.5 reflects a sample of the telephone volume by day of week for a sample medical practice. From these data, we learn that more staff are needed to work the telephones on Monday, tapering off throughout the week. This is not at all surprising for most medical practices; inbound telephone demand is often highest on Mondays. The key to staffing the telephones is to staff for this work variability in call demand, not simply create a static staffing model that is the same throughout the entire week, regardless of inbound telephone call volume.

EXHIBIT 5.5 INBOUND TELEPHONE VOLUME BY DAY OF WEEK

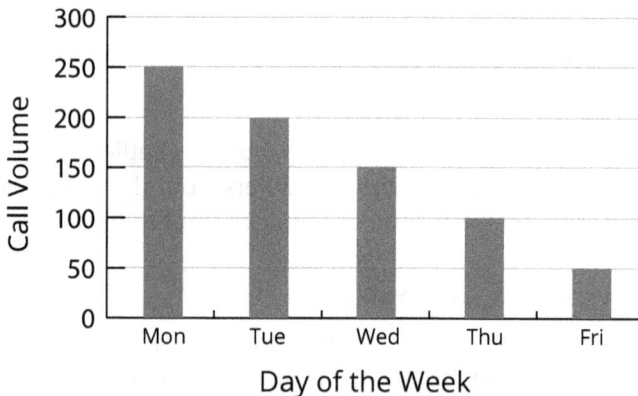

Next, graph the inbound telephone calls by time of day. In Exhibit 5.6, we can see that the inbound telephone call volume also varies by time of day. Calls at our sample medical practice are at their highest volume from 8:00 a.m. to 12:00 p.m. each day.

In fact, approximately 70% of the calls are received in the morning between these hours. Thus, we learn from these data that more staffing resources need to be deployed in the morning than in the afternoon, again suggesting the use of a flexible rather than static staffing model to manage the inbound telephone demand.

EXHIBIT 5.6 INBOUND CALLS BY TIME OF DAY

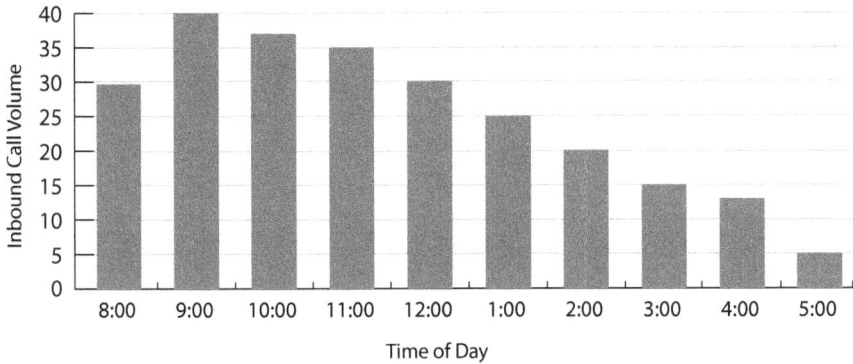

A further refinement to the staffing model can be made by linking both measures we have examined thus far: inbound telephone calls by day of week and by time of day. For example, you may find that your call volume is highest on Monday mornings between 8:00 a.m. and 10:00 a.m. Additional refinements can be made for seasonality (for example, flu season) and other variations, such as an increase in call volume two days after patient statements are mailed or after recall notices are transmitted via the portal. In this fashion, you can anticipate and appropriately staff for the volume of work to be performed.

Beyond the volume of inbound calls by day of week and time of day, the reason for a call also provides us with information to appropriately staff the telephones. The purpose of the calls is important because we may staff differently by call type. Furthermore, when we learn the reasons for inbound calls we can work to reduce inbound call demand by better anticipating patient needs. Ask staff to collect these data for a one-week representative period. Discuss the importance of capturing accurate data. The data may not be perfect because it is difficult to collect the data during a day in the life of a medical practice; however, this collection of data will provide important information to help you optimally staff your telephones.

The graph of the inbound calls by reason for call for our sample medical practice is provided in Exhibit 5.7. As demonstrated by this graph, the highest call volume is for scheduling, followed by clinical calls. The third highest call volume is for medications and prescription renewals.

EXHIBIT 5.7 INBOUND CALLS BY REASON FOR CALL

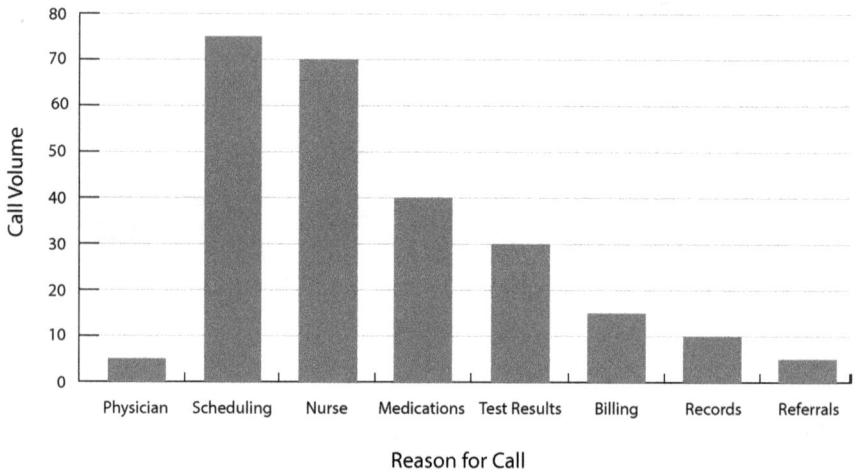

These data provide additional information to develop the staffing model for our sample medical practice. We now have an approximation of the volume of calls for nurse triage and the volume of calls for appointment scheduling and other patient inquiries.

In Exhibit 5.8, we report the inbound telephone volume by day of the week that we computed earlier in this chapter. We then identify the type of inbound call by using the percentages that we obtained based on the analysis of the reason for the inbound calls. Our sample medical practice highlights clinical calls, scheduling calls, and all other calls (the latter is assumed to involve message-taking).

EXHIBIT 5.8 INBOUND CALLS BY DAY OF WEEK AND REASON FOR CALL

	Mon	Tue	Wed	Thu	Fri
Total Inbound Calls	250	200	150	100	50
Clinical Calls (30% of total)	75	60	45	30	15
Scheduling (28% of total)	70	56	42	28	14
Messages (42% of total)	105	84	63	42	21

3. Evaluate Staff Workload Ranges

To build the staffing model for telephone management in our sample medical practice, identify the expected staff productivity workload ranges for telephone work. These were reported in Chapter 4, Staff Productivity, and are restated in Exhibit 5.9 for nonclinical calls. For clinical calls, staffing expectations for nurse triage/advice via telephone or via portal is 65 to 85 per day, as reported in Chapter 4, Exhibit 4.3.

EXHIBIT 5.9 PRODUCTIVITY EXPECTATIONS FOR COMMUNICATIONS[3]

Work Function	Per Day	Per Hour
Telephones with messaging	300-500	42-71
Telephones with routing (electronic system) only	1,000-1,200	142-171
Appointment scheduling with mini-registration	75-125	11-18
Appointment scheduling with full registration	50-75	7-11

As we discuss in Chapter 4, Staff Productivity, it is important to make sure that the expected workload ranges are consistent with your medical practice. For purposes of this example, let's assume the midpoint of each of the applicable expected staff workload ranges is selected as the targeted production level for the staff, as follows:

Telephone nurse triage:	75 calls per day
Patient scheduling, mini-registration:	100 calls per day
Telephone messaging:	400 calls per day

4. Calculate Required Staff FTE

Calculate the staff FTE required to manage the inbound telephone demand if these targeted production levels are met. In our sample medical practice, we assume that medical practice leaders decided to have a nurse triage unit manage clinical calls and a patient scheduling unit manage administrative calls.

We use the call data from our sample medical practice to build the required staffing FTE levels by dividing the call volume by the expected work level for each type of call to calculate the required staff FTEs to manage the work volume.

This calculation is demonstrated in Exhibit 5.10 for our sample medical practice. For example, on Monday:

- 75 clinical calls are received. The expected productivity for telephone nurse triage in this practice is 75. Dividing 75 by 75, we calculate 1.00 staff FTE to manage the clinical call volume.

- 70 scheduling calls are received. The expected productivity for scheduling in this practice is 100 calls. Dividing 70 by 100, we calculate 0.70 staff FTE to manage the scheduling call volume.

- 105 calls require message-taking. The expected productivity for messaging for this practice is 400 calls. Dividing 105 by 400, we calculate 0.26 staff FTE to manage the message-taking calls.

We continue this approach for each day of the week and each type of call.

EXHIBIT 5.10 REQUIRED STAFF FTE TO MANAGE INBOUND TELEPHONES BY DAY OF WEEK

	Mon	Tue	Wed	Thu	Fri
Total inbound calls	250	200	150	100	50
Clinical Calls	75	60	45	30	15
Expected productivity	75	75	75	75	75
Total Required Clinical FTE	**1.00**	**0.80**	**0.60**	**0.40**	**0.20**
Scheduling Calls	70	56	42	28	14
Expected productivity	100	100	100	100	100
Required staff FTE	0.70	0.56	0.42	0.28	0.14
Message Calls	105	84	63	42	21
Expected productivity	400	400	400	400	400
Required staff FTE	0.26	0.21	0.16	0.11	0.05
Total Required Scheduling/Message FTE	**0.96**	**0.77**	**0.58**	**0.39**	**0.19**

5. Perform a Gap Analysis

Once you have benchmarked your communications staff and have analyzed and built your staffing model based on work productivity, assess the gaps, comparing current staffing levels with those suggested by the productivity model you have built. For this sample practice, if no changes are made to inbound call demand, we need to create a flexible staffing model rather than a static model to optimize staffing for the work consistent with the variability in inbound telephone demand by day of week.

Further refine the staffing model by applying the same steps to the call data based on time of day. For example, you may find that the volume of inbound calls is highest in the morning, from 8:00 a.m. to 10:00 a.m., gradually declining until 1:00 p.m., when there is a second peak in call demand. Follow the same steps outlined earlier; however, refine the analysis by time of day in addition to day of week.

Be sure to adjust your staffing model over time based on feedback from other performance measures. For example, if call abandonment rates are higher than baseline, the staffing model may need modification. Similarly, if a new physician is hired who generates a significant increase in inbound telephone demand, an adjustment to the staffing model may be needed. A staffing model is not static; regularly evaluate and update it consistent with the changing needs of your medical practice.

INNOVATIVE STAFFING STRATEGIES FOR COMMUNICATIONS

Staffing for the work is critical, however, this is an opportune time to redesign the work itself. Determine the best work process for your medical practice and design a flexible staffing model around the type of work and quantity of work to be performed. Let's now turn to some key areas to address as you deploy communications staff in your practice.

REDESIGN WORK PROCESSES

The most innovative process for communications management is to replace the telephone altogether. The telephone requires synchronous communication between two parties (the caller and the responder, in most cases, that of a practice staff member). Determine if technology can provide an alternate communications platform. A portal or other secure electronic platform can replace a portion of inbound telephone calls by allowing patients to self-schedule, receive test results, request prescriptions, and message their physician without telephoning the practice. While these strategies will never replace the telephone, they can certainly have a positive influence over it.

> THE MOST INNOVATIVE PROCESS FOR COMMUNICATIONS MANAGEMENT IS TO REPLACE THE TELEPHONE WITH A SECURE ELECTRONIC PLATFORM THAT FACILITATES PATIENT SELF-SERVICE.

CLINICAL CALLS

Explore the many alternatives that can be used to manage clinical calls, then determine the best process for your practice. Options include:

- Take messages by telephone operators and route the message to the nurse, who then places an outbound call to subsequently reach the patient.

- Transfer the caller directly to the nurse; if the nurse is not available, a message is taken.

- Provide a portal or other secure electronic platform for patients to message the physician (or nurse); depending on the clinical circumstances, the physician or nurse uses the portal to message the patient back — or places an outbound call to subsequently reach the patient.

- Design the portal or other secure electronic platform to handle a distinct portion of clinical calls; for example, notification of normal test results and patients' prescription renewal requests are routed through and managed via the portal.

ADMINISTRATIVE CALLS

Determine your preferred work process for administrative, nonclinical calls. Options include:

- Assign staff who reside in the front office to also manage inbound calls.

- Designate the responsibility of managing inbound calls to one employee — or one function (for example, check-out).

- Establish a call center to manage all inbound calls or just a portion of them (for example, only scheduling calls).

- Process certain administrative tasks via the portal or other secure electronic platform; for example, requests for referrals or scheduling, and appointment confirmations.

- Provide a secure electronic platform for patients to 'self-serve,' in contrast to placing an inbound call; for example, permit self-scheduling.

The work process you select for each type of call — clinical or administrative — determines the staffing volume and skill mix of staff needed to manage inbound communications in your medical practice. It also impacts practice efficiency and the timeliness by which patients can access your practice. This decision also says volumes about whether your medical practice is a group practice where resources are shared among physicians via a care team or a collection of individual practices, with limited resource sharing.

CREATE A FLEXIBLE STAFFING MODEL

Recognize the fluctuations in the volume of communications by day of week, time of day, and reason. Flexibly delegate the appropriate number of staff and skill mix of the staff consistent with the work.

Based on the example provided earlier in this chapter, if there is no change to inbound telephone call volume, our sample medical practice needs the following staffing model:

Monday
1.00 staff FTE clinical support staff and 1.00 staff FTE telephone scheduler, a total of 2.00 staff FTE for all inbound communications.

Tuesday and Wednesday
The 2.00 staff FTE communications staff can be assigned a significant amount of other work to be performed during the day, since a 1.00 staff FTE designation for each of the types of calls is not warranted based on the work.

Thursday and Friday
A different staffing strategy for communications is warranted. For example, one clinical support staff can be assigned to manage the full inbound telephone volume (rather than a mix of scheduling and clinical staff); this staff member should also be delegated significant other roles and responsibilities on Friday.

As technology is adopted by your practice, as well as your patients, alter your staffing model, to include changing your staffing ratios, as warranted. For example, as more patients utilize the portal to obtain information, inbound telephone volume may decline, permitting a reduction in staff FTE levels deployed to communications management. Since the operations and work environment of a medical practice are constantly changing, be flexible in your staffing model. We discuss flexible staffing strategies in Chapter 11, Teleworking and Flexible Staffing.

> As technology is adopted by your practice and your patients, alter your staffing model and staffing ratios, as warranted.

Designate Staff Dedicated to Communications

Take telephones off stage and manage them separately from the face-to-face interaction with patients:

- Deploy front office staff to manage either patient check-in/check-out or the telephones, not both, and
- Deploy clinical support staff to manage the patient flow process during the visit (visit preparation, retrieval, vital signs, rooming, assisting) or the telephones and portal, not both processes simultaneously.

This staffing model permits the telephones and portal to be managed in real time, reducing the need for extensive message-taking. It also provides more immediate feedback to patients in response to their needs.

Achieve First-Call Resolution

Failure to act on an initial request creates a deluge of inbound calls. Patients simply will not wait for days — and, often, just for hours — for a response, resulting in patients often placing multiple inbound calls to check on the status of their initial inquiry. Therefore, first-call resolution — responding to inquiries in real time — is an excellent method to control demand.

First-call resolution is best accomplished by promoting the use of a secure electronic platform for patients to utilize for non-urgent communication. This permits the practice to prioritize and process the electronic messages in a nonsynchronous manner between tasks, as time allows. Regardless of the communications platform, adopt clinical protocols, as appropriate, to allow the workflow to be performed more efficiently and effectively. Encourage patients to self-serve via offerings provided on a secure electronic platform.

Even with technology enhancements, medical practices will continue to receive telephone calls. Better-performing medical practices manage these calls in one step by responding to the patient in real time, achieving first-call resolution by:

- Staffing for the work,
- Separating the work of patient flow from communications,
- Deploying technology,
- Making a commitment to resolving the requestor's needs upon the initial request, and
- Anticipating follow-up questions the patient may have and proactively provide information at the initial call, reducing the volume of subsequent calls.

REDUCE INBOUND COMMUNICATIONS DEMAND

Contemplate the calls that may have been avoidable in the first place. These could encompass issues ranging from office hours (which could, instead, be posted on your website or stated on your telephone hold message) to patients' questions about their care that could have been better managed in the exam room (for example, "What was that medication you told me to take?").

Once you capture the reason for the inbound communications to your practice, act to reduce that demand. Exhibit 5.11 outlines steps you can take to reduce inbound demand.

If you are successful in reducing the volume of inbound communications, revisit your staffing model. It may be possible to reduce the number of staff devoted to telephone or portal management and/or delegate additional responsibilities to these staff if their work volume declines.

EXHIBIT 5.11 ACTIONS TO REDUCE INBOUND
COMMUNICATIONS[4]

Type of Inbound Communication	Action
Scheduling	Offer self-scheduling Utilize appointment recall Make post-operative appointments at the time of surgery scheduling Proactively manage care transitions; follow up with patients post-discharge and post-emergency department visit
Test results	Set realistic expectations with patients regarding the timeframe of notification Provide negative test results via the portal Give patients a take-home tool that outlines how they will learn of their test results, to include registering for and locating results on the portal Create a closed-loop process to ensure the tests are administered, the results are received and reviewed, and patients are notified of results Give patients a top-five list of questions and answers specific to their visit, thereby anticipating patient needs
Prescriptions and medications	Perform electronic prescribing Accept prescription renewal requests via the portal; alert patients to proceed to the pharmacy when a refill(s) exists Ask patients if they need a renewal during their visit Execute clinical protocols Deploy clinical decision support tools to recognize payer formularies upon prescribing Automate prescription monitoring with state database, if applicable
General information	Forward callers to an automated line that details directions to the practice in languages appropriate for the patient population; include public transportation if applicable Place information about the practice on Website, portal and social media

KEY QUESTIONS TO ADDRESS

Today's medical practice must staff not only the telephones, but also each of the varied communication channels and technologies offered to patients, referring physicians and the public. Address the following key questions as you staff for communications management:

- What is the volume of inbound calls, secure messages, and portal inquiries by day of week and time of day?

- What is the workload of each staff member involved in telephone and portal management?

- Why are patients calling? Can a portion of calls be prevented by improving the communication to the requestor?

- Can we consolidate work? For example, can one nurse (or a small nurse unit) manage the inbound calls and secure electronic messages for physicians rather than reside this work with each nurse?

- Will cross-training of staff permit us to improve communications during high peak demand?

- What improvements to our telephone management can be made to permit the call to be managed in one step involving first-call resolution?

- What steps can we take to minimize inbound calls? For example, can electronic access methods for patients be expanded and/or can the medical practice better anticipate patients' inquiries, thereby preventing an inbound telephone call?

- What action can we take to more effectively integrate staff who manage non-office communications on the care team?

- Can we improve or expand the functionality of existing technology, or add new opportunities? For example, can we convert appointments from online requests to self-scheduling appointments?

SUMMARY

In this chapter, we share performance expectations for communications management. We build the staffing model for communications by analyzing the volume and reason for inbound communications and applying expected staff workload ranges to align staff with the work. We then explore work redesign options, to include alternative communication platforms that enable first-call resolution, promoting innovative staffing strategies for communications management.

ENDNOTES

1 Woodcock, Elizabeth W. and Deborah Walker Keegan. 2018. Patient Access: Tools and Strategies for the Medical Practice, Englewood, Colo.: Medical Group Management Association. Reprinted with permission.

2 Ibid.

3 Ibid.

4 Ibid.

CHAPTER 6

STAFFING THE FRONT OFFICE

Y our front office staff represent the first in-person contact a patient has with your medical practice. As such, these staff members serve not only as customer service representatives, but also as marketers, flow masters, and practice billers. This multifaceted role is challenging and requires a skill set that stretches between high interpersonal acumen and analytical skills. More and more, medical practices are recognizing that these staff are the key to patient access and satisfaction, as well as practice efficiency and profitability.

In this chapter, we:

- Describe key work functions for the front office
- Provide front office performance expectations
- Build the staffing model for front office work
- Share innovative staffing strategies for the front office
- Provide key questions to address for staffing the front office

KEY FRONT OFFICE WORK FUNCTIONS

Key work functions for front office staff include patient financial clearance, reception and check-in, and patient check-out. The detailed work involved in each of these work functions is described in the following section.

> FRONT OFFICE STAFF MUST POSSESS A SKILL SET THAT STRETCHES FROM HIGH INTERPERSONAL ACUMEN TO ANALYTICAL ABILITY.

THE PATIENT FINANCIAL CLEARANCE/PRE-VISIT PROCESS

Patient financial clearance is one of the key functions in today's reimbursement environment. Financial accountability is on the rise with a significant portion of patients holding insurance that features a high cost share, increasing patients' out-of-pocket payments, to include copayment, coinsurance and deductibles.

Patient financial clearance involves each of the steps necessary for the business of medicine to be accurately conducted. This work is now typically performed prior to patients arriving for their scheduled visits and includes insurance verification, eligibility verification, demographic verification, understanding of payment history, time-of-service payment determination, and ensuring referrals are obtained prior to services performed. Authorizations may also be within the scope of the front office but are often performed in the business office.

The Patient Reception and Check-in Process

Patient reception and check-in typically involves the following tasks:

- Receive the patient with a warm greeting,
- Capture, verify and enter patient demographic and insurance information,
- Collect time-of-service payments, post payments to the system and issue receipts,
- Obtain signatures as required by the practice in compliance with state and federal regulations, for example, Health Insurance Portability and Accountability Act (HIPAA) notification,
- Scan insurance cards for new patients, patients with an insurance change, and patients who received new cards from their health plan (even if not an insurance change), and verify insurance and benefits eligibility,
- Take photographs of new patients for their account in the electronic health record (EHR) system, if applicable, and
- As a final step, arrive patients in the EHR system.

The check-in staff may schedule the next appointment at check-in (for example, well-child exam or follow-up chemotherapy treatment), anticipating the follow-up appointment that is needed, however, this is more commonly handled at check-out. Check-in staff also conduct cash balancing at the end of the day, with attention to internal controls and security of cash, checks, and credit and debit cards.

> THE FRONT OFFICE STAFF LARGELY DETERMINE WHETHER A CLEAN CLAIM IS SUBMITTED TO PAYERS.

THE PATIENT CHECK-OUT PROCESS

At check-out, the staff member acts based on the follow-up instructions in the patient's record in the EHR system (although some practices continue to utilize paper orders).

Check-out staff typically conduct the following tasks:

- Schedule patient follow-up appointments, appointments for imaging, laboratory, and other ancillary services, and consultations with specialists,

- Process outbound referrals, and

- Confirm visit charges and work pre-adjudication claim edits.

These tasks often vary greatly by medical practices. Some practices choose to incorporate the tasks within the exam room at the end of the clinical encounter.

Evaluate each of these work functions and determine the work scope appropriate for your front office staff. Specify the who, what, when, where, and how the task is to be performed as part of your staffing deployment model.

FRONT OFFICE PERFORMANCE EXPECTATIONS

The skills needed for the front office service encounter include high interpersonal communication, customer-focused decision-making, problem solving, initiative, judgment, compassion, and high energy. Add to that the necessities of today's medical practice — knowledge of payer requirements, how to determine patient responsibility payments, when to obtain referrals, how to determine coordination of benefits, and other similar highly complex business-of-medicine issues — and it is clear the front office requires sophisticated members on the care team to skillfully and efficiently execute tasks. Consistent with that sophistication, we expect a level of performance and contribution from these staff far greater than in the past.

Institute performance expectations for front office staff and measure your staff's ability to achieve these standards. Exhibit 6.1 outlines common expectations regarding front office work to get you started.

Exhibit 6.1 Performance Expectations for Front Office[1]

- **Patient Financial Clearance**
  - » Registration errors are less than 2% of claim edits and claim denials[2]
  - » All referrals are obtained prior to the visit
  - » The medical practice knows the amount to be collected at the time of service for each patient
- **Patient Reception and Check-In**
  - » Every patient is greeted warmly, with eye contact; use of the patient's name is encouraged if possible
  - » Patients are not asked to repeat information that has already been provided
  - » Insurance coverage is verified 100% of the time
  - » Scanning of insurance cards takes place at each visit (or based on established practice protocols)
  - » New patients are photographed for their account in the EHR system (based on established practice protocols)
  - » Required signatures are collected 100% of the time
  - » Copayments are collected 98% of the time[3]
  - » Co-insurance, deductibles, and patient responsibility balances are collected 75% of the time[4]
  - » A receipt is provided to every patient who makes a payment, regardless of the amount
- **Patient Check-Out**
  - » Follow-up appointments include the reasons for the follow-up visits
  - » Patients are provided with information and tools so they know next steps and do not have to "go fish" for information after their visit
  - » Subsequent visits, specialty consultations, procedures and tests are scheduled consistent with physician orders
  - » Referral processes are completed to permit transition of patient to specialist or to procedure
  - » If applicable, charges are reviewed for accuracy, with claim edits due to charge entry errors less than 2% of charges entered[5]
  - » Missing charges are queried daily to ensure 100% of services are captured and billed

> TODAY'S FRONT OFFICE IS COMPLEX, REQUIRING SOPHISTICATED
> MEMBERS ON THE TEAM; WE EXPECT A LEVEL OF PERFORMANCE AND
> CONTRIBUTION FAR GREATER THAN THE PAST.

BUILDING THE FRONT OFFICE STAFFING MODEL

To build the staffing model for front office work, proceed through the following steps.

STAFF BENCHMARKING ANALYSIS

Benchmark the staff involved in front office work, following the approach we describe in Chapter 3, Staff Benchmarking. The MGMA survey staff category of *total front office staff* and its work function level of *medical receptionists* typically are used for this benchmarking analysis.

STAFF PRODUCTIVITY ANALYSIS

Follow the steps described in Chapter 4, Staff Productivity, and outlined herein, to evaluate the productivity levels of your front office staff.

1. Determine the Unit of Work

Identify the arrived patient volume (as opposed to the volume of patients reported on the scheduling template), which is the unit of work for patient check-in, with typically the same volume attributed to patient check-out. The number of referrals to be processed is the unit of work for referral management staff.

2. Capture Data

Collect a representative work sample. Determine the patient arrived visit volume for a one-week period by day of week and session per day. Do not select a peak volume period for this sample. The goal is to staff for the typical work volume and then use other techniques to manage peak volume demand.

Exhibit 6.2 reports data for a sample medical practice. It reflects arrived patient visits for each day of the week for each session of the day.

EXHIBIT 6.2 ARRIVED PATIENT VOLUME BY DAY OF WEEK AND SESSION PER DAY

	Mon	Tue	Wed	Thu	Fri
Morning Arrived Visits	50	45	40	60	25
Afternoon Arrived Visits	70	50	45	55	5

3. Evaluate Staff Workload Ranges

Exhibit 6.3 outlines the productivity expectations of the front office staff to utilize in this analysis (a restatement of Exhibit 4.2 provided earlier in this book). Evaluate these expected staff workload ranges to determine if they are consistent with your medical practice. For example, can your staff be reasonably expected to conduct patient check-in at a volume of 100 to 130 per day, the equivalent 14 to 19 per hour (assuming they are asked to perform data verification only)?

EXHIBIT 6.3 PRODUCTIVITY EXPECTATIONS FOR FRONT OFFICE[6]

Work Function	Per Day	Per Hour
Pre-visit or on-site financial clearance	60–80	9-11
Patient check-in -With data verification only -With data verification and cashiering	100-130 75-100	14-19 11-14
Check-out -With scheduling and cashiering -With scheduling, cashiering, charge entry	70-90 60-80	10-13 9-11
Referrals (inbound or outbound)	70–90	10–13

Source: Walker Keegan, Deborah and Elizabeth W. Woodcock. 2106 The Physician Billing Process: Navigating Potholes on the Road to Getting Paid. Englewood, Colo.: Medical Group Management Association. Reprinted with permission.

4. Calculate Required FTE

Calculate the required FTE by dividing the actual work volume by the expected workload level, as depicted in Exhibit 6.4. For example, in our sample practice on Monday morning, 1.11 staff FTE are required to check in the morning arrived visit volume, decreasing to 0.56 staff FTE on Friday morning. When both check-in and check-out work functions are evaluated, a total of 2.54 staff FTE is required on Monday morning, decreasing to 1.27 staff FTE on Friday morning.

EXHIBIT 6.4 REQUIRED STAFF FTE FOR PATIENT CHECK-IN AND CHECK-OUT (INCLUDING CHARGE REVIEW)

	Mon	Tue	Wed	Thu	Fri
Morning Arrived Visits	50	45	40	60	25
FTE staff required for check-in	1.11	1.00	0.89	1.33	0.56
FTE staff required for check-out	1.43	1.29	1.14	1.71	0.71
Total FTE Staff Required AM	**2.54**	**2.29**	**2.03**	**3.04**	**1.27**
Afternoon Arrived Visits	70	50	45	55	5
FTE staff required for check-in	1.56	1.11	1.00	1.22	0.11
FTE staff required for check-out	2.00	1.43	1.29	1.57	0.14
Total FTE Staff Required PM	**3.56**	**2.54**	**2.29**	**2.79**	**0.25**

Notes: Staff workload expectation for patient check-in and cashiering: 75 to 100 per day; 90 used in above table (45 each half-day clinic session).

Staff workload expectation for patient check-out, scheduling, and charge review: 60 to 80 per day; 70 used in above table (35 each half-day clinic session).

From Exhibit 6.4, we learn that a range of 1.27 to 3.04 staff FTE are required to manage the morning clinic session and 0.25 to 3.56 staff FTE are required to manage the afternoon clinic session, depending on the day of the week.

Note the wide variability by day of week and session per day. A further differentiation based on hours within each session can also be computed.

Consistent with one of the recurring themes of this book, a medical practice needs to staff for the work. Therefore, if this medical practice is not able to have a consistent volume across the week or otherwise reduce its patient visit variation, its staffing deployment model should be flexible based on day of week and session per day consistent with the work. If a flexible model is not adopted, then the medical practice will not be staffed at optimal levels. Depending on clinic session per day, it will have either too many or too few staff needed to conduct the work.

5. Perform a Gap Analysis

Once you have benchmarked your front office staff and have analyzed their productivity in comparison to expected productivity levels, analyze the gaps. Work to understand why your staffing model may be different from industry norms.

For medical practices with referral management activity, the unit of work is the number of referrals to be processed. Exhibit 6.3 outlines the expectation related to work quantity for referral management staff. We typically expect referral processors to manage 70 to 90 inbound and/or outbound referrals per day, which is the workload equivalent of 10 to 13 per hour. The work of referral management generally includes contact with referring physicians, payers and patients; processing the required electronic forms; securing (and following up to obtain) approval; scheduling appointments; and submitting the appropriate referrals. The referral tasks depend on whether the referral is an inbound referral requiring acceptance by the practice, or whether it is an outbound referral processed on behalf of a patient who is being referred to another provider. Furthermore, the specific requirements vary by payer.

INNOVATIVE STAFFING STRATEGIES FOR THE FRONT OFFICE

Staffing for the work is critical, however, it is an opportune time to redesign the work itself. With newer technologies, there is no need to continue to manage the patient check-in and check-out processes in the traditional in-person, sequential pattern.

Redesign Work Processes

Evaluate the following work redesign and staffing innovations and determine if one or more are applicable for your medical practice. Importantly, with technology it may be possible to delegate work to patients who can self-serve and conduct some work functions that have traditionally be performed by front office staff.[7]

The following two examples describe work process redesign and the impact it has on the staffing model.

Patient Reception and Check-in

Traditional Process: The patient travels to a check-in desk, queuing in a line and waiting for the next available staff representative. The patient may make multiple trips to the front office, for example, the patient may be asked to complete forms and bring them back up to the desk when completed or be asked to sign in and sit down and be called back up to check in.

Redesigned Process: Optimize pre-visit tasks and ask patients to self-arrive at a kiosk or via a tablet. Perform other check-in functions when the patient is in the exam room.

Procedure Scheduling

Traditional Process: The patient is required to walk to the check-out area or scheduling desk, wait in a queue, and have a face-to-face meeting with the scheduler.

Redesigned Process: Designate a scheduler to travel to the patient while in the exam room, processing the work on a tablet or send the patient home and call or securely message the patient at a subsequent time.

Below are additional work redesign and staffing innovation strategies, with many emphasizing a patient-centric approach. We encourage you to evaluate their applicability for your medical practice. If the decision is made to implement one or more of these work processes, revisit your staffing model to make sure you have the correct number and type of staff required for the newly redesigned work.

PATIENT FINANCIAL CLEARANCE

Self Pre-register

Establish an automated method for pre-registration. Deploy standalone functionality or incorporate the task in the portal. Allow registration forms to be completed by patients prior to the visit, incorporating data and signatures via an interface to the practice management and EHR systems.

Conduct Real-time Eligibility

Automate the insurance verification process for your medical practice by deploying real-time insurance verification and benefits eligibility. The function should be accessed via the practice management system so that it may be performed seamlessly during the workflows related to scheduling and arrival. If the eligibility fails, staff can intervene immediately with patients to determine alternate coverage.

Collect Payments

Communicate with patients to provide price estimates for upcoming non-emergent, scheduled procedures and surgeries. Before or after the service, collect payments online via the portal or payment on file solution, thereby minimizing this work at the front office and business office, and ensuring payment. In addition, consider collecting patient balances at the time of appointment reminders, thereby reducing this work function at patient check-in.

Deploy Price Estimation Tools

Deploy price estimation tools to support the accuracy and timelines of collection. Offer online bill payment.

PATIENT RECEPTION AND CHECK-IN

Eliminate the Queue

Eliminate waiting and queuing and bring the work to the patient. Room the patient at the time of arrival and perform the registration process while the patient is in the exam room using a tablet.

Create a Flexible Staffing Model

Do not staff solely based on peak periods. Create notification/alert systems (like a grocery store when a line at the check-out area begins to form). Cross-train staff to work in multiple areas.

Adopt Patient Self Check-in

Implement kiosks or tablets for patient check-in, thereby delegating work to the patient, who can perform this function electronically at your medical practice.

Stagger Visit Start Times

By staggering appointment times for physicians (for example, one physician starts at 8:00 a.m., another starts at 8:15 a.m., and so forth), the staff can attend to the full scope of work for each patient, which is often difficult to accomplish with large numbers of patients arriving at the same time for appointments. Some medical practices have templates that feature top-of-the-hour appointments, which creates boluses of patients requiring service. Stagger the start time of clinics and avoid templates that feature patient appointments only at the top and bottom of each hour.

PATIENT CHECK-OUT

Eliminate the Queue

Eradicate waiting and queuing, and bring the work to the patient. Ask clinical staff to schedule follow-up appointments and procedures while the patient is in the exam room and/or have schedulers travel to the exam room to interact with patients and eliminate the check-out desk. Workstations on wheels with a computer or tablet help facilitate the workflow.

Co-locate Staff

Locate check-in and check-out staff adjacent to one another, and cross-train them so they can assist each other during peak periods. For example, if the first patient is scheduled at 8:00 a.m., there will not be any patients to check out until approximately 8:30 a.m. Staff can be assigned to help with check-in during that 30-minute period. Use tablets situated on mobile workstations to move into the reception area; or push back the chairs in the front office and have all staff stand during this time so they can be optimally effective in these dual roles.

Advocate for Patients

Designate staff as financial advocates to help patients understand their insurance plans and their personal financial obligations — and ensure that your practice is paid in a timely fashion.

Do Not Batch Work

Process work throughout the day rather than wait until end of day, thereby improving staff efficiency. Waiting is a form of batching and delaying the work.[8]

Delegate Additional Work Functions

Delegate tasks such as sorting and opening mail (and other similar episodic work functions), to be completed by front office staff during downtime.

Consolidate Referral Processing

Centralize referral workflow with a single staff member or unit, rather than each staff member conducting this function. This creates work efficiencies and frees up staff to attend to other important work functions.

> PERMIT PATIENTS TO SELF-PRE-REGISTER AND SELF-CHECK-IN.
> ERADICATE WAITING AND QUEUING AND BRING WORK TO THE
> PATIENT IN THE EXAM ROOM.

Each of the above work redesign options impacts the staffing model of a medical practice. Evaluate new technologies, redesign your work processes and then revisit your staffing model to ensure you are optimally staffing for the work.

KEY QUESTIONS TO ADDRESS

As you staff your front office, consider the following key questions:

- What steps can we take to prepare business functions in advance of the visit?
- What steps can we take to reduce variable work levels for the staff? Can visit times be staggered to reduce work variation?
- Is there work that patients can conduct online that will streamline their visit experience?
- Can work steps be combined rather than continue with process handoffs between staff?
- Can work accuracy be improved by employing a different

staffing model?

- Is there an opportunity to centralize work functions such as referral management?
- Can we create more efficient work processes through automation?

SUMMARY

In today's medical practices, there are fewer and fewer human touches with the patient. Patients can access information and appointments via the practice's portal, and they may communicate through secure messaging in between their face-to-face visits with the physician. With less interpersonal interaction, we need to make sure that the ones patients do have matter.

Your front office staff are the visible representation of your medical practice. Their work is critical, not only for financial viability, but also for patient access and service delivery. In this chapter, we describe the key work functions of front office staff, how to build a successful staffing deployment model for the front office, and innovative work redesign and staffing strategies that can take your medical practice to the next level of performance.

ENDNOTES

1 Walker Keegan, Deborah L. and Elizabeth W. Woodcock. 2016. The Physician Billing Process: Navigating Potholes on the Road to Getting Paid. Englewood Colo.: Medical Group Management Association.

2 Ibid.

3 Ibid.

4 Ibid.

5 Ibid.

6 Ibid.

7 For more front office strategies, see Woodcock, Elizabeth W. 2018. Front Office Success: How to Satisfy Patients and Boost the Bottom Line. Englewood, Colo.: Medical Group Management Association.

8 Woodcock, Elizabeth W. 2014. Mastering Patient Flow. Englewood, Colo.: Medical Group Management Association.

CHAPTER 7

STAFFING THE ENCOUNTER

The clinical support staff are those care team members who interact with the physician and patient to deliver patient care whether that is provided via a traditional face-to-face visit or newer delivery systems, such as patient portal or telemedicine. Determining the right combination of registered nurses (RNs), licensed practical nurses (LPNs), and medical assistants (MAs) for the work and delegating appropriate work are critical if we are to optimize their contribution to the care team.

In this chapter, we:

- Describe key clinical support staff work functions
- Build a clinical support staff model to form the foundation of the care team
- Share innovative strategies for deploying clinical staff
- Share new roles and responsibilities for clinical support
- Provide key questions to address in the development of the clinical staffing model

KEY CLINICAL SUPPORT STAFF WORK FUNCTIONS

Clinical support staff are deployed in support of the clinical care of the patient, to include managing and coordinating clinical issues that arise before, during and after an encounter with the physician.[1] Clinical support staff are generally assigned to 1) support the face-to-face encounter, 2) respond to patients' communications, to include telephone triage and advice and secure, electronic messaging, and 3) support care coordination via case management and/or population health via panel management. Each of these work functions is further described in the following sections.

PATIENT ENCOUNTER SUPPORT

We expect clinical staff who support the face-to-face patient encounter to anticipate both physician and patient needs and actively participate in the visit itself.

Work functions delegated to these staff include:

- *Pre-visit clinical preparation.* Anticipate patient, visit, exam room, and procedure needs, and identify outstanding clinical needs of patients, for example, via clinical decision support or a registry.

- *Patient flow support.* Retrieve patient, take vital signs, obtain medication history, obtain reason for visit, prepare patient for the exam, assist with the visit, obtain Advance Beneficiary Notice (ABN) (if applicable, at the time of service), and keep the physician on time.

- *Procedure support.* Anticipate needs of physician and patient for procedures, participate in procedures, administer injections and immunizations, and conduct nursing visits, such as blood pressure checks, allergy shots, complex wound care management, and other similar nursing encounters.

- *Patient discharge support.* Educate patients, discharge patients from the exam room, schedule and/or arrange for follow-up procedures and tests, review charges for completion, and obtain medication pre-authorizations.

These workflow decisions may be impacted based on compliance with state regulations regarding scope of practice, and, if applicable, facility or payer-imposed standards of care.

> CLINICAL SUPPORT STAFF ARE DEPLOYED IN SUPPORT OF THE CLINICAL CARE OF THE PATIENT, TO INCLUDE MANAGING AND COORDINATING CLINICAL ISSUES THAT ARISE BEFORE, DURING AND AFTER THE ENCOUNTER.

CLINICAL COMMUNICATIONS

As we discuss in Chapter 5, Staffing Communications, a nurse triage and advice unit to manage inbound and outbound calls and messages is an efficient staffing model for communications management — and it reduces the time to respond to patient telephone inquiries and secure, electronic messages, since staff are fully devoted to this function.

Key roles and responsibilities for nurses assigned to manage clinical communications include:

- Respond to inbound patient communication about clinical issues as received via telephone calls and secure, electronic messages,

- Assess patients' chief complaints to determine plan of care, to include scheduling an appointment, and

- Place outbound calls and secure, electronic messages as directed by physician, for example, test results, post-operative care and medication changes, and provide follow-up instruction to patients.

The nurses assigned to manage clinical communications may also be involved in obtaining medication pre-authorizations, screening incoming correspondence (to include test results and consult notes), and providing advice to internal staff who have questions. Furthermore, tasks are assigned to these nurses by physicians and advanced practice providers via the EHR system, necessitating attention to the task work queue throughout the day.

CASE AND PANEL MANAGEMENT

More and more, medical practices are identifying a specific staff member(s) to manage case management and panel management and/or serve as health coaches to promote patient self-management. These roles typically involve a significant amount of outbound communication (for example, "Ms. Smith, you are due for your mammogram. Please schedule yours.").

Key roles and responsibilities for nurses assigned to manage care and panel management include:

- Coordinate transitions of care, to include working with patients who have been recently discharged from the hospital or emergency department,

- Manage and work patient registries to identify patients for recommended preventive and follow-up care, for example, mammography screening and Pap smears,

- Engage in partnership with patients to help them manage

chronic disease, for example, congestive heart failure and chronic obstructive pulmonary disease, and/or

- Evaluate patient population and conduct panel management consistent with targeted quality metrics.

Some medical practices rotate nurses through these roles to ensure that each is cross-trained and has work variety.

Building a Clinical Staff Support Model

Follow the steps outlined in this section to develop a successful clinical staff support model.

Staff Benchmarking Analysis

To determine whether you have the correct number and skill mix of clinical staff, first benchmark these staff to the available survey instruments. In this fashion, a medical practice can determine if it has a skill mix consistent with peer practices in the same specialty.

As outlined in Chapter 3, Staff Benchmarking, benchmarks are available not only at the level of the specific clinical staff position of RN, LPN, and MA, but also at the categorical level of total clinical support staff (which combines each of the three positions). This assessment allows you to compare your practice with similar practices on two levels: 1) the total number of clinical staffing support (regardless of skill mix or licensure of these staff) and 2) the specific mix of RNs, LPNs, and MAs to determine whether there is staffing opportunity. You may also want to benchmark the cost of staff in this category to determine if your clinical support staff costs are in line with peer practices.

Staff Productivity Analysis

Follow the steps outlined in Chapter 4, Staff Productivity, and outlined herein, to identify the correct number and skill mix/licensure of staff for your practice.

1. Determine the Unit of Work

Recognize the unit of work for clinical support staff, which varies based on the work they are tasked to perform.

- For staff involved in patient flow support, the unit of work is the volume of arrived patient visits and the type of support to be provided for the visit.

- For staff involved in clinical communications, the unit of work is the volume of inbound telephone calls and secure, electronic messages.

- For staff serving as panel managers and health and wellness coaches, the unit of work is the number and type of patients assigned.

There may be other work for which to account, to include remote care encounters.

The unit of work designation for key work assignments is depicted in Exhibit 7.1.

EXHIBIT 7.1 UNIT OF WORK DESIGNATION

Work Assignment	Unit of Work
Patient flow support	Encounter volume and type
Nurse triage and advice	Volume of inbound clinical telephone calls and secure, electronic messages
Panel management	Active patient count. This may be a cohort of patients, such as those from a particular risk-based arrangement with a health plan or accountable care organization or a provider's full panel.
Care management	Number of cases assigned for care outreach. This is typically a specific cohort of patients, such as those with congestive heart failure or other disease.

Note that medical practices may differ in their unit of work designation. As an example, some highly productive medical practices identify the exam room itself as the unit of work for clinical staff assigned to patient flow support, rather than the number of encounters. Instead of adopting the encounter as the unit of work, they staff the exam room. Each medical assistant (or other clinical support staff, depending on work delegation) is assigned a specific exam room. His or her job is to room the patient, support the visit — including assisting with the exam and functioning as a scribe for the physician — and discharge the patient from the exam room. This process is repeated throughout the day. The clinical support staff recognize the importance of maintaining the flow of patients, and filling and turning over exam rooms to facilitate high patient volumes.

2. Capture Data

Identify the number of work units for a representative one-week period. Measure these workloads based on day of week and session per day. As examples, capture:

- Arrived patient visit volume for clinical staff involved in the encounter,

- Number of inbound clinical telephone calls and secure messages for   staff involved in communications management and nurse triage, and

- Panel counts and/or assigned patients for clinical staff involved in case management and panel management.

3. Evaluate Staff Workload Ranges

Evaluate the expected staff productivity workload ranges and determine their applicability for your practice. The expected workload range for clinical support staff is reported in Exhibit 7.2 (a restatement of Exhibit 4.3 of this book). Note that these ranges are generally broad, because the specific type of patient, as well as the clinical intervention, dictates the amount of time required for the clinical staff.

EXHIBIT 7.2 PRODUCTIVITY EXPECTATIONS FOR CLINICAL SUPPORT[2]

Work Function	Per Day	Per Hour
Nurse triage/advice via telephone or portal*	65-85	8-12
Patient intake: patient rooming, vital signs	Variable based on specific work that work can be delegated; typically, 25 to 40 patients per day	N/A
Visit support: nurse visit support, procedures, education	Variable based on specific work that can be delegated; typically, 25 to 40 patients per day	N/A
Panel management; health and wellness coaching	Variable, based on type and breadth of services provided. See Chapter 9: Staffing for Value-Based Care for a detailed discussion	N/A

N/A = not applicable

Note: The expected staff workload range assumes full nurse triage and advice, not simply prescription renewals or responding to inquiries of a nonclinical nature, such as scheduling or information requests.

*Source: Woodcock, Elizabeth W. and Deborah Walker Keegan, 2018. Patient Access: Tools and Strategies for the Medical Practice, Englewood, CO, MGMA. Reprinted with permission.

The productivity ranges for many of the clinical support work functions depend on delegated work scope. In these instances, develop staff productivity ranges specific to your medical practice by meeting with staff to discuss the time it takes to complete each key task or observing staff during their work.

4. Calculate Required Staff FTE

Based on your current work volume, calculate the number of staff full-time equivalent (FTE) required for the work by dividing your current work volume by the volume of work you expect your staff to perform. As an example, if there are 250 clinical calls on Monday and the lowest end of the productivity workload range of 65 per day as reported in Exhibit 7.2 is applicable for your medical practice, divide 250 by 65 to calculate 3.85 staff FTE required for this work.

5. Perform a Gap Analysis

Compare this built clinical staff model with your current model and perform a gap analysis, asking and answering critical questions regarding your model.

INNOVATIVE STAFFING STRATEGIES FOR CLINICAL SUPPORT

Let's now turn to some key areas to address in your clinical staffing model to include innovative strategies for deploying clinical support staff in your medical practice.

DETERMINE WORK SCOPE

The traditional nursing roles in the medical practice are expanding. New roles for nurses include care management, panel management, guided self-care, and other patient outreach and coaching activities to assist patients, each involving heightened engagement of clinical support staff on the care team. Clinical staff are assisted in this work via new technologies, to include the practice's registry, as well as the clinical decision support tools embedded in the practice's EHR system.

Determine the scope of work to be performed by your clinical staff. For example:

- What clinical preparation is expected of the clinical support staff?
- What rooming and vital signs are expected to be performed?
- What level of autonomy does the nurse have in ordering, responding to patient inquiries via the telephone and portal, and other similar tasks?
- What role are the staff expected to play in support of the physician and the patient in between face-to-face visits?
- How is the nurse engaged with clinical decision tools in the EHR system?
- How can we adjust workflow and assignments so that everyone is working to the top of their license?

- What role do the clinical support staff play in e-consults and e-visits?
- What role do the clinical support staff play in secure, electronic messaging between the patient and care team?

Asking probing questions like these assists in identifying the optimal work scope for the clinical support staff. Let's examine two case studies to demonstrate this approach toward analyzing work scope.

CASE STUDY A: A WHOLE LOT OF NURSES

This pediatric practice has five physicians. Each physician is assigned a 1.00 FTE LPN and there is also a shared 1.00 FTE RN who administers shots, for a total of 6.00 FTE clinical support staff. To determine if this model is appropriate, ask and answer the following questions:

- Does each physician require clinical support staff to assist during clinic 10 sessions per week? If not, how many sessions require assistance?
- How many patients does each physician see?
- What type of work do the LPNs perform?
- Do the LPNs manage both the patient flow process and the telephone/messaging process?
- Are LPNs required for each of the work functions?
- Are LPNs performing any nurse visits?
- How many shots are administered by the RN?
- What is the distribution of shots by day of week and time of day?
- Who is performing the sight and hearing exams for well-child checks?
- Is there a lab? If so, who is performing the blood draws and processing the specimens?
- Who is preparing and tracking immunizations?
- Since the assignment is by physician, do the LPNs support one another as a team, to include covering when one of them is absent from work?

- Are the workstations efficient? Could a mobile workstation on wheels improve the efficiency of the clinical support staff and/or physicians?
- What are the barriers to efficient workflow?
- Are staff members working to the top of their licenses?
- What is the scope of practice for an RN, LPN and MA in the state in which the practice is located?
- What work functions could be delegated to a medical assistant or another staff member?

CASE STUDY B: DR. GREEN ON THE PHONE

Dr. Green is routinely interrupted to respond to clinical inquiries from patients and physicians. Analysis of the time spent handling telephone calls and secure electronic messages is 10 minutes each hour (80 minutes per day).

To determine if a change to the clinical support model will improve the physician's efficiency and productivity, ask and answer the following questions:

- What types of telephone calls and messages are received?
- What is the turnaround time required for these communications?
- Can a clinical staff member manage some or each of the communications?
- What roles are the nurses performing in the medical practice? Can they assume the role of communications management for some or each of these calls and messages?
- Could the creation and adoption of clinical protocols assist in delegating work to a nurse(s)?
- Is first-call resolution embraced? Are patients and referring physicians calling repeatedly to get a response?
- Could inbound communications from patients and referring physicians be bifurcated to improve handling of each type of communication? For example, patient inquiries could be first triaged by a nurse, with the physician as the first responder to referring physician calls.

- Is the patient's care managed over the telephone and portal because there is no appointment availability? If so, could a nurse be designated for nurse visits and patients be seen in the practice or via remote care instead of managed via the telephone and portal?

- How can we improve our communications with patients? For example, if some of the calls are patients inquiring about their upcoming procedures, how can we address these issues during the patient's visit – and reduce inbound call volume?

- What is the opportunity cost of the physician in managing the telephone calls? For example, is the physician seeing lower patient visit volumes due to this workflow? What is the cost per visit of the physician's time?

Identify your current clinical staffing deployment model, perform a gap analysis regarding work quantity, and ask probing questions regarding your model so you can identify opportunities to improve the clinical staffing model for your practice.

CREATE A CARE TEAM MODEL

As you build your staffing model for the encounter, determine whether you can strengthen your care team model. That is, instead of each physician being assigned one medical assistant or nurse who does everything in support of the patient visit and the communications directly attributed to each physician, determine if a shared resource can be allocated. Viewing your clinical staffing model from the lens of the patient is a useful tactic to help link resources in support of the work.

As examples:

- A designated nurse or triage unit handles telephone calls and secure, electronic messages rather than assign this work to each physician's nurse or medical assistant,

- If physicians are not working 10 sessions per week in the clinic, re-deploy clinical support staff to assist other physicians and/ or be flexibly scheduled not to work,

- Assign medical assistants to manage patient flow, with a triage unit managing the phones and portal and a team nurse assisting with procedures, injections, wound care, and other similar nursing duties, and

- Align staff to support care teams. These are teams of physicians and advanced practice providers who work together. The collaborative effort often includes a staff member assigned to panel management or health coaching. The tasks may include, but are not limited to, transitions of care, preventive care, and care coordination. Historically, these functions may have not been performed, or fell onto the physician's nurse to conduct when he or she was able.

Regardless of whether a care team model is emphasized by your medical practice, it is not physically possible for a single nurse to provide patient flow and visit support for 30 patients, while also managing 100 calls and messages in a single day in a timely and accurate fashion. Identify clinical staff to manage patient flow and visit support and separate clinical staff to manage patient communications. In this fashion, the staff can be fully devoted to these roles rather than attempt to manage both processes simultaneously.

> IT IS NOT PHYSICALLY POSSIBLE FOR A SINGLE NURSE TO TIMELY AND ACCURATELY PROVIDE PATIENT FLOW AND VISIT SUPPORT FOR 30 PATIENT VISITS WHILE ALSO MANAGING 100 CALLS AND MESSAGES. ASSIGN CLINICAL STAFF TO SUPPORT PATIENT FLOW OR COMMUNICATIONS, NOT BOTH SIMULTANEOUSLY.

EVALUATE CLINICAL STAFF SKILL MIX

What is the best mix of clinical support staff involving RNs, LPNs, and MAs in a medical practice? The answer to that question is: It depends. It is contingent on a host of issues, including:

- Role delegation by the physician,
- The specialty of the medical practice's physicians,
- The type of patients presenting to the medical practice,
- The state's scope of practice requirements, and
- The local job market and the availability of specific types of staff.

Consistent with the themes in this book, we need to staff for the work. We also seek to deploy staff wisely, positioning staff to work at the top of their licensure.

To determine if your practice is managing to the top of licensure of its clinical support staff, consider the following exercise. On separate sticky notes, list each task of the clinical support staff. So, for example, there is a note for patient rooming, another note for patient vital signs, and so forth. On a large wall in your office or conference room, place column headers of RN, LPN, MA and Other. Then place each of the sticky notes under the header that accurately matches the licensure required for the specific task. Exhibit 7.3 depicts this approach to analyzing skill mix needs.

When this exercise is conducted, you may find that you have an opportunity to re-assign work and/or change your staffing model consistent with the work. As examples:

- If your licensed nurses are rooming patients and this can be conducted by a medical assistant, determine if changes to work assignment or staff skill mix are warranted, and

- If you are staffed with registered nurses with each responsible for inbound clinical communications, evaluate whether a consolidated nurse triage unit can be formed, thereby limiting the number of licensed clinical staff and altering the skill mix of the practice's overall clinical support team.

Exhibit 7.3 Clinical Support Staff Skill Mix Exercise

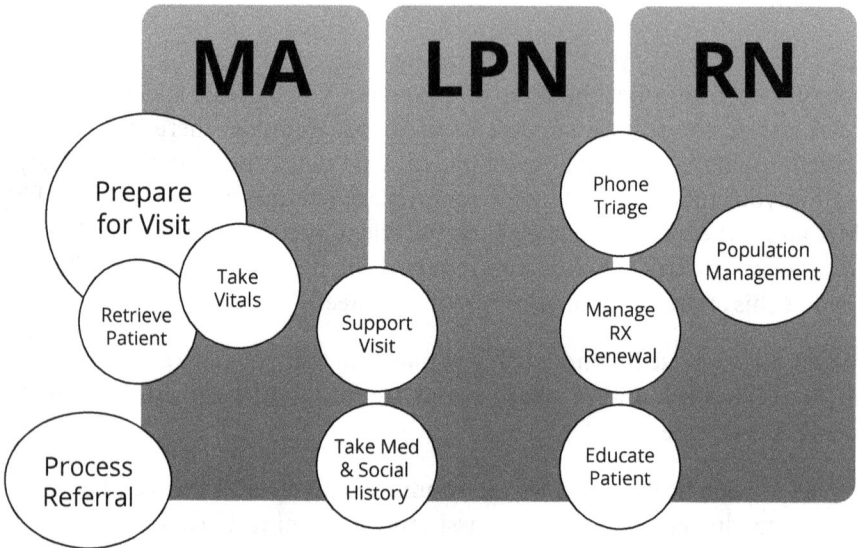

The goal is to deploy clinical support staff so they function at the top of their licensure when possible. This depends on state law in terms of work delegation to each licensee based on the scope of practice outlined by the state. Below is an example of the types of work that are being delegated to clinical support staff. Note these are only examples. As the clinical staffing model is formulated, evaluate your state law to determine any applicable scope of practice requirements.

Medical Assistants

- Pre-visit planning
- Disease registry entry
- Medication reconciliation

Licensed Practical Nurses

- Nurse visits within scope of practice and licensure

- Education and coaching
- Care transition management

Registered Nurses

- Assistance with managing complex illness (under supervision and within scope of licensure)
- Triage and advice
- Education and coaching
- Population management

CLINICALLY PREPARE FOR THE VISIT

With EHR systems, new staff roles and tasks are required to prepare for the patient visit. Deploy staff to review registries or clinical decision support systems, ensure orders completion and verify test results in preparation for the visit, along with preparing for next steps in the patient's care and treatment plan.

The history, background, and referral records for new patients must also be entered in the electronic record. Determine the best work process and staffing model for this process, which can involve medical records staff, scheduling staff, clinical support staff or delegated to the patient (with an upload of his or her data to the electronic record). Regardless of who is delegated this responsibility, establish a goal of populating the EHR in advance of the physician-patient encounter so the physician has the information needed to make the initial visit with the patient meaningful.

CONDUCT CLINICAL INTAKE

Conduct a detailed assessment of the rooming and intake process to determine the role for the clinical support staff. Consider the clinical needs of the physician, available technologies, and the tasks that support the appropriate choice of the level of the evaluation and management (E/M) visit code.

As an example, patients may be given a tablet when they arrive for their visit.

- The patient confirms insurance and demographic information, as well as his or her past family, social and medical history on the tablet.

- The patient delivers the tablet to the front office. A front office staff member queues the patient-documented information in the EHR system.

- The nurse introduces his or herself, escorts the patient to the exam room, indicating the actions that will be taken during intake to keep the patient informed. The data gathered from the patient is referenced; the nurse confirms (or revises) and documents the patient's past family, social, and medical history.

- The nurse reviews historical and current medications, using a list of medications (including dosage) on records imported from the pharmacy into the EHR system. Medication reconciliation may be completed now or readied for the physician to finalize upon his or her arrival, with medications updated from a drop-down menu of options, with reasons provided for discontinuation of medications as appropriate.

- Vitals are taken, with the respective devices, such as blood pressure, height and weight and are interfaced directly with the EHR system.

- Alerts from the clinical decision support tool are highlighted, as appropriate.

- Standing orders, if applicable, are reviewed and acted upon.

- The nurse reviews the information gathered and documented, departs the exam room, and communicates to the physician that the intake is complete.

The elements of the intake vary by physician, specialty, scope of practice, and internal protocols, however, the key is leveraging technology and the clinical support staff in a role that promotes the efficiency and effectiveness of the physician in performing the exam, assessing the patient, and creating a plan of care. Following the provider-patient visit, the clinical support staff may also return to the exam room, after the creation of the plan, to provide education and support, schedule follow-up testing and perform other required activities prior to discharging the patient from the exam room.

> LEVERAGE CLINICAL SUPPORT STAFF IN A ROLE THAT PROMOTES THE
> EFFICIENCY AND EFFECTIVENESS OF THE PHYSICIAN.

COMPLETE EHR TASKS

In an EHR system, the inbox of tasks and messages expands and contracts daily; managing EHR tasks is an issue of work delegation and accountability. Determine the best staffing support strategy as well as performance expectations regarding the accuracy and timeliness of this work.

- For inboxes assigned to clinical support staff, determine if this work (or specific types of tasks) can be consolidated in the medical practice with a focused group of staff, rather than be assigned to each individual clinical support staff member. This permits focused attention and typically results in improvements in work efficiency and timeliness.

- For physician inboxes, determine the best work process and staffing model for your practice:

  - The physician works the full inbox alone,

  - The nurse first works the inbox and flags items for the physician, or

  - There is a shared inbox involving the physician and nurse, with the physician huddling with the nurse at established intervals during the day to jointly work the tasks.

Address this decision and the appropriate staffing strategy as part of your ongoing EHR system management.

SUPPORT THE PATIENT-FACING VISIT

When staffing the patient-facing visit, evaluate the role of the clinical support staff. Their role depends both on your specialty and the delegated authority granted to these staff:

- Some of your clinical support staff may be in the exam room for the total visit with the provider, for example, actively assisting with the exam or a procedure.

- Others may room and ready the patient for the provider, coming into the exam room during the visit to assist only when requested, for example, to administer an injection or immunization, provide education, or schedule follow-up tests.

There is no single industry standard for their role, which is why we have recommended managing to the top of licensure when possible.

Importantly, with EHR systems, evaluate whether the patient visit needs to continue to consist of a set of sequential steps: the patient interacts with a nurse, then the physician in sequence. Instead, concurrent steps to the visit can be taken. For example, the physician and the nurse can enter the exam room together, with the nurse documenting the exam based on the physician's oral reports, assisting with the visit, and providing end of visit education and discharge instructions. This collaborative physician-nurse encounter model typically requires a new clinical staffing model for a medical practice.

> WITH EHR SYSTEMS, A COLLABORATIVE VISIT MODEL MAY BE ADOPTED RATHER THAN A SEQUENTIAL VISIT MODEL, REQUIRING CHANGES TO YOUR CLINICAL STAFFING MODEL.

DETERMINE REMOTE CARE SUPPORT

Assign staff to provide remote care support, to include:

- Scheduling e-consults,
- Responding to secure messages, and
- Setting up telemedicine-based visits.

The work involved in supporting remote care cannot simply be piled higher and higher on the staff involved in the face-to-face patient visit. Instead, a formal staffing plan and a deployment model are required. This involves redistributing work tasks, roles, and responsibilities to effectively staff for this work. We discuss additional staffing strategies for remote care support in Chapter 9, Staffing for Value-Based Care.

ENHANCE INTERNAL COMMUNICATIONS

Your staff members who provide clinical support to the encounter operate in busy, often unpredictable environments where communications between the physician and staff member or among co-workers must be optimized. Rather than require the provider to go look for the nurse or the nurse to wait until the provider comes out of the exam room to communicate, implement techniques (based on your practice, its facility, and its technology resources) to enhance internal communications and provider and staff efficiency. Evaluate the following internal communication strategies for your practice.

- *Team huddle.* A morning huddle before the clinic begins to review the day ahead to include who is scheduled, the reasons for visits, and the preparation that has already been conducted and that which remains. Medical practices engaged in performance improvement also reflect on mistakes made the day prior to avoid those in the future.

- *Visible signals.* Flags, lights, or other visible signals regarding the state of the exam room; the flag may indicate the presence of a certain type of staff member or provider (for example, green flag or light indicates the patient is being roomed by the medical assistant) or the readiness (for example, red may signal that the physician should enter the room next).

- *Devices.* Communication devices that can be worn on the person; wireless ear buds or headsets connected to a communication device can be helpful for some staff members, particularly if movement is required, allowing the staff member to still be available for an incoming communication or instruction; smartphone apps can also fill this role. Particularly if staff members and/or providers work outside of the office, such a communications system can be vital. Another strategy is the use of instant or direct messaging, often a feature embedded in the practice management or EHR system. Security of the devices and their transmission, however, is paramount.

- *Patient tracking.* Patient tracking from arrival to departure via an EHR system. Although the function is often driven by manual input, high-performing practices determine the protocol for tracking as well as its usage; this includes steps to take if a patient has been at any one step for too long. Beyond the time devoted to each step in the patient flow process, overall patient time in the practice, known as patient cycle time, is also tracked.

- **EHR system communication.** Enhanced communication capabilities afforded an EHR system, to include:
  - ⊚ the orders feature (as the order signals the action step for the patient), which often needs assistance by a staff member, such as scheduling a test,
  - ⊚ a separate referral feature, which may also incorporate the action,
  - ⊚ the clinical decision support feature (as the alert indicates an action that is recommended for the patient's care), and
  - ⊚ the task feature, which allows messages to be taken, routed, saved and closed in the system.

- **Other communications technologies**
  - ⊚ Radiofrequency identification (RFID) technology, or another sophisticated tracking system, offers an alternative solution. Like any system, it requires attention to detail in its adoption and execution.
  - ⊚ Overhead pagers and speaker phones offer another option, however, many practices find these are distracting and adversely impact the patient experience.

As this list demonstrates, there are many options to enhance internal communications between providers and employees to improve efficiency and effectiveness. Investigate technologies and select the option that is best for your practice. To be effective, everyone in the practice must use the features in a consistent manner, and protocols should be established for their use. For example, performance expectations may include that EHR system inbox tasks must be resolved within 24 hours, documentation must be complete and accurate, and the task must be closed on completion.

Changing Roles of Clinical Support Staff

When analyzing work scope of your clinical staff, recognize the changing role of these staff due to EHR systems and value-based care requirements and take these into account as you redesign your clinical support staff model. Many of these changes are summarized in Exhibit 7.4 and a detailed discussion is provided in Chapter 9, Staffing for Value-Based Care.

As this list demonstrates, changes in roles involving physician instruction, patient inquiries, proactive care management, and test and laboratory results reporting are a direct result of technology. Importantly, they also impact the clinical support staffing model.

Exhibit 7.4 Changing Role of Clinical Support Staff

Separation of internal and external patient visit support	Telephone nurse/portal support is separate from patient visit support
Physician instruction to nurse	Instant messaging or inbox message to nurse
Physician/nurse instruction to patient	Electronic message to patient
Patient inquiries	Patient navigator to provide access and care assistance; inquiries maintained in running lists and proactively managed with patient; use of visuals (charts and graphs) to assist patient self-management and activation
Proactive care management	Care manager coordinates care outside of patient-facing visits; registries and clinical protocols managed by nurse and physician with patient self-management and reporting
Procedure and test results	Electronic patient recall; patient self-serve results via portal
Documentation	Scribes; expanded nurse charting roles involving structured data

We explore three of these roles in greater detail on the next page.

Patient Navigator

Some medical practices have introduced patient navigators to support patients in accessing the practice and providing pre- and post-encounter support. There are generally three different patient navigator types.

1. **Resource Patient Navigator.** The patient navigator provides information and resources to patients and their families. This may include educating to community resources, resolving patients' access questions, and other resource-based questions.

2. **New Patient Navigator.** Patient navigators work with new patients to ensure streamlined patient access and smooth entry to the practice, making sure the patient is scheduled for the right physician, ensuring a timely appointment, handling referrals, managing the financial pre-visit process, and holding discussions with the patient regarding their visit itinerary. These navigators will typically receive calls from patients regarding questions and concerns and the navigators put the patients in touch with the correct area of the practice, as appropriate.

3. **Clinical Patient Navigator.** A clinical patient navigator (typically a licensed nurse) is assigned to each patient to manage the patient's course of care. The care and treatment plan, test results, etc. are routinely reviewed by this navigator. Patients typically meet the nurse navigator on a frequent basis while in the clinic, for example, every second or third visit, and may receive telephone calls or secure messages (for example, care outreach) from the nurse to check on their status. Mobile health devices are often deployed with instructions regarding transmitting the data to the navigator to allow an ongoing assessment of patients' conditions.

Two primary keys to success of each of these models are to 1) clearly define the roles, responsibilities and role boundaries of this position and 2) ensure back-up coverage. If a physician's nurse is designated as the nurse navigator, for example, and he or she is off on Friday and assisting the physician in clinic on Monday, a patient's telephone call from Friday may only be responded to many days later. Thus, back-up coverage for these roles is a prerequisite.

CARE MANAGER

A care manager is another relatively new staffing role for many medical practices. Care managers perform tasks typically targeted to a specific patient cohort. The assignments vary based on specialty but are often in accordance with the needs of complex patients, or those with specific clinical issues.

Key roles and responsibilities for a care manager include:

- Obtain special certifications and/or training for the designated patient population,
- Coordinate care delivery for the cohort of patients,
- Monitor high-risk patients; intervene as clinically appropriate,
- Preview appointment schedules and identify patient issues pertinent to the patient visit,
- Engage with clinical decision support tools,
- Manage consultations, referrals and transfers of care to other providers and facilities, for example, home health, and
- Perform patient coaching and face-to-face nursing visits, as needed.

For some practices, the designated nurse in this role may serve the entire practice. This is common in a primary care practice that serves as a medical home for its patients. The title of this role varies — case manager, panel manager, health coach and nurse care coordinator, for example — but the key is the nurse serving in a proactive role in caring for the needs of the patient population. Instead of being reactive — picking up the phone when a patient calls for advice or assisting the physician with patients who present for face-to-face encounters — the nurse in this role is proactive. Using tools such as a registry and the EHR's clinical decision support, the nurse reaches out to patients to manage their care. This role is critical for a practice to successfully execute and deliver population health.

For other practices, only a small cohort of patients may be managed by the care manager. This may include, for example, patients with congestive heart failure or those who need transitions of care, such as a patient to be discharged from the hospital to a skilled nursing facility. EHR systems have permitted medical practices to transition from a "build it and they will come" mentality to a patient outreach mentality. In these practices, clinical staff are assigned to work via electronic registries and recall systems to reach out to patients in a care or case management role. This helps the patient comply with his or her care and treatment plan. It also reduces inbound telephone calls, inappropriate admissions, and inappropriate visits. Instead, a nurse reaches out to patients to determine their status and responds to their questions and concerns. More formal programs involving this type of outreach use health and wellness coaches to work with groups of patients based on diagnosis or type of intervention, such as recent hospital discharge.

Regardless of whether the care manager is managing a patient population or a specific patient cohort, we expect to see this staff member serving as an integral member of the care team.

SCRIBES

EHR systems permit consolidated storage of patient information and enhanced access to data and information for care and treatment, yet they often are also found to slow down a busy physician. In these situations, scribes are often introduced to document key aspects of the patient visit. A recent study documented a 41 percent to 66 percent decrease in the time the physician spent completing documentation when scribes are used in the primary care setting.[3]

Scribes are particularly value-added for physicians who rely on specific measurements or other detailed data that require documentation. As examples:

- A dermatologist conducts a full-body exam on a patient with a scribe recording the size and location of suspicious skin anomalies for future monitoring, and

- An ophthalmologist examines patients using various equipment with a scribe recording the physician's verbal account of findings.

More and more medical practices use scribes (with some designating nurses or medical assistants to these roles) to improve physician efficiency. Some are also using "virtual scribes" who are not physically present in the exam room but participate via technology.

Key Questions to Address

As you develop your clinical staffing model, ask and answer the following key questions:

- What work functions have been delegated to each of our clinical support staff members?

- How does our clinical support staff volume compare with available benchmarks in similar practices? What is the skill mix of the benchmarks in comparison to the medical practice?

- What steps are taken to prepare for the visit (for example, EHR system alerts, registries, exam room preparation, patient preparation, procedure preparation)? Is additional visit preparation needed?

- How are our patient telephone calls and secure electronic messages related to clinical issues managed? What are the reasons for the communications and what is the current turnaround time to respond to the patient?

- Are staff members working to the top of their license? What work functions could be more appropriately delegated?

- Can sharing of staff in a group practice model improve work scope and focus our clinical staff on discrete work functions?

- Are there other staffing deployment models that may better meet our physicians' and/or our patients' needs?

- What communication channels can we develop to improve provider-clinical staff and practice-patient communication?

- Will a newer delivery model involving expanded work delegation and managing to the top of licensure help us transition to personal, value-based care?

SUMMARY

In this chapter, we discuss how to analyze and build a clinical staff model for your medical practice. We also share innovative staffing strategies used in many of today's medical practices, to include new roles and responsibilities of the clinical care team due to EHR systems and value-based care requirements. By deploying clinical support staff to support the face-to-face encounter and a separate set of staff focused on communications, we can structure a workforce that can support the physician and the patient as part of a well-coordinated care team.

ENDNOTES

1 For purposes of simplicity, in this chapter we cite support to the "physician." Clinical support staff may also support advanced practice providers and other rendering providers.

2 Woodcock, Elizabeth W. and Deborah Walker Keegan, 2018. Patient Access: Tools and Strategies for the Medical Practice, Englewood, Colo.: Medical Group Management Association. Reprinted with permission.

3 Rocco DiSanto and Venkat Prasad. Scribe Utilization in the Primary Care Environment. Journal of Medical Practice Management, July/August 2017. Vol 33. No 1. pp 66-70.

CHAPTER 8

STAFFING THE BUSINESS OFFICE

Innovation in billing is on the horizon: picture a model where the patient swipes a card upon departing your practice. Data are directly submitted from your management information systems to the payer, with the payer transferring money to your bank account in real-time. The residual financial accountability is then debited from the patient's credit card, which is already on file; the balance is zero and receipts are issued through secure electronic means. When that time comes, it will truly revolutionize the staffing strategy used for billing and collection work.

Until then, however, correctly staffing for the multitude of challenges that practices encounter in getting paid is essential. We are faced with a convoluted and complex revenue cycle that requires an optimal staffing plan.

In this chapter, we:

- Present key business office work functions
- Build the staffing model for the business office
- Share innovative staffing strategies for the business office
- Discuss staffing for consumer-directed health plans
- Discuss staffing for value-based reimbursement
- Provide key questions to address for business office staffing

KEY BUSINESS OFFICE WORK FUNCTIONS

The work involved in billing and collections is typically divided into front-end billing and back-end billing functions.

FRONT-END BILLING

Front-end billing functions include the following key areas:

- Credentialing
- Registration and scheduling
- Patient financial clearance

- Patient reception and check-in
- Patient check-out
- Referrals and pre-authorizations
- Coding
- Charge capture and submission
- Financial counseling
- Payment at the time of service

Some of these functions — coding and charge entry, for example, may largely be automated. In Chapter 6, Staffing the Front Office, we discuss the work functions related to patient financial clearance, patient reception and check-in, and patient check-out, and how to build a successful staffing model for this work.

BACK-END BILLING

Back-end billing work functions are those that are typically performed in a business office. The work includes:

- Claim submission and claim edits
- Accounts receivable follow-up
- Patient collections
- Statement submission
- Payment and denial posting
- Credit and refund management
- Payment variance analysis
- Denial posting and resolution
- Reporting results and data analysis

BUILDING THE STAFFING MODEL FOR THE BUSINESS OFFICE

To build the staffing model for your business office, follow the same steps we present in earlier chapters of this book.

STAFF BENCHMARKING ANALYSIS

Benchmarks are reported for patient accounting staff at the functional level in the MGMA survey instruments. These staff are a subset of the total business operations staff category. Per MGMA, patient accounting staff are defined as "billing and collections staff, such as department supervisor, billing/accounts receivable manager, coding, charge entry, insurance, billing, collections, payment posting, refund, adjustment, and cashiering staff."[1] Follow the staff benchmarking process described in Chapter 3, Staff Benchmarking, to benchmark staff FTEs and cost of business office staff.

STAFF PRODUCTIVITY ANALYSIS

Use Chapter 4, Staff Productivity as a guide to evaluate current staff productivity and compare it to expected staff workload ranges for each key billing function, as described herein.

1. Determine the Unit of Work

Recognize the units of work for the business office; these may vary depending on the specific function that has been tasked to the staff to perform. For example, the unit of work for account representatives is the number of accounts or invoices to be followed and worked. The unit of work for denial management is the number of denials to be investigated and appealed or adjusted, as appropriate.

2. Capture Data

Capture data for the specific work tasks assigned to the staff. For example, capture the volume of claims submitted, the number of accounts to be followed up, the number of denials to be managed, and so forth.

3. Evaluate Staff Workload Ranges

Staff productivity workload ranges are available for key billing functions of the revenue cycle, some of which are reported in Exhibit 8.1 (a restatement of Exhibit 4.4). Evaluate these ranges to determine their applicability to your medical practice. Importantly, determine which specific level within the range to target when building your staffing model.[2]

Exhibit 8.1 Productivity Expectations for the Business Office[3]

Work Function	Per Day	Per Hour
Credits researched and processed	60–80	9-11
Insurance follow-up and action	50-70	7-10
Patient follow-up and action	70-90	10-13

Source: Walker Keegan, Deborah and Elizabeth W. Woodcock. 2016. The Physician Billing Process: Navigating Potholes on the Road to Getting Paid. Englewood, Colo.: Medical Group Management Association. Reprinted with permission.

The "Potholes" book contains additional expected staff workload ranges related to billing; the above exhibit reports a subset of this data.

Many factors influence the ability of staff to work within these ranges. These include the leverage of technology, the practice management and electronic health record (EHR) systems, the tools and processes required of the staff, the age and complexity of the accounts, and other similar factors. When issues of quantity versus quality arise, it is recommended that quality be the primary focus when identifying staff workload and performance.

4. Calculate Required Staff FTE

Calculate the required staff FTE for the specific work task under analysis. As examples:

- *Credits researched and processed.* Let's assume the lowest end of the workload range is appropriate for your practice, with a staff member able to research and process 60 credits per day or 9 per hour. If 100 credits per day need to be worked, calculate the required staff FTE for this work by dividing 100 by 60, to arrive at 1.67 staff FTE.

- *Insurance account follow-up and action.* As another example, let's assume that your practice needs to follow-up on 250 invoices per day. Let's also assume that a single staff member working full-time on this work function is expected to work

50 invoices or 7 per hour (the lowest end of the staff workload range for insurance account follow-up). The work of 250 invoices will require 5.00 staff FTE (calculated as 250 divided by 50).

5. Perform a Gap Analysis

Analyze the gaps between your current staffing levels and those suggested by the benchmarks and productivity levels and identify areas of opportunity to improve your business office staffing model.

INNOVATIVE STAFFING STRATEGIES FOR THE BUSINESS OFFICE

Although it is important to staff for the work, it is also critical to evaluate the work and determine if redesign is warranted. We devoted an entire book to the revenue cycle and we encourage readers who seek to redesign their business office staffing models to review that text.[4] Some key staffing innovation highlights are presented below.

EVALUATE FRONT-END BILLING PERFORMANCE

Assess your front-end billing staff model. Capture data to evaluate the performance associated with front-end billing, to include:

- Rejections due to registration and other front-end errors,
- Claim denials due to deductible, incorrect payer, lack of referral authorization, ineligibility, and non-covered services,
- Claim denials due to coding, and
- Charge submission lag time.

Use these data as a guide to determine the magnitude of performance opportunity you have and determine if a change to your staffing model is warranted. Many better-performing medical practices cite evidence that their investment in improving front-end billing staffing and education has paid off, with higher percentages of clean claims being submitted and paid by payers. Doing it right the first-time results in better cash flow – and fewer staffing resources being deployed for back-end billing functions and rework.

ORGANIZE INSURANCE ACCOUNT FOLLOW-UP BY PAYER

Organize insurance follow-up staff by payer to permit early identification of reimbursement delays and to increase staff efficiency when working account follow-up and denial management. Each payer has its own rules and requirements related to coding and bundling, payment policies, and other important factors. So, for example, we recommend a staff member (or staffing unit) dedicated to Medicare, another dedicated to Medicaid, another dedicated to your key commercial payers, and so forth.

Depending on the claim volume and complexity, the staffing delineation may include a blend of payer and service line. For example, within the insurance account follow-up unit, there may be account follow-up staff devoted to Medicare and then divided by service line (such as cardiovascular). This permits work delegation consistent with payer and specialty-specific knowledge.

ENSURE EQUITABLE WORK DISTRIBUTION

Traditionally, insurance account follow-up has been assigned to various employees based on work volume. For example, if five staff members are assigned to this work, each has been delegated approximately 20 percent of the work. Recognize that each payer demands a different level of work. As an example, Workers' Compensation claims are more complex and time consuming than Medicare claims. Similarly, following up on outstanding government claims is typically easier than commercial claims, given the government's standardized requirements and processes. Ensure an equitable distribution of work among staff by considering the difficulty of the work associated with each payer.

LINK COMPLEMENTARY WORK FUNCTIONS

Integrate work areas by function to build a broader breadth and scope of responsibility for your staff. This model also minimizes work handoffs and improves staffing efficiency. For example, the tasks of payment posting (which is now largely automated) and account follow-up can be integrated:

- Both tasks require in-depth, payer-specific knowledge to recognize and manage services that are not paid, or those that are paid incorrectly.

- Each task requires the staff to comprehend and interpret the information the payer is conveying through its reason and remark codes.

Since both the payment posters and account follow-up staff require this same knowledge, consider adopting total account ownership (TAO), which focuses the work of payment posting and insurance account follow-up with one individual responsible for a specific payer who is well versed in its nuances.[5] The staff member assigned to Medicare, for example, manages the entire reimbursement process from that payer, from the receipt of the remittances to the final payment. Care must be taken from an internal controls perspective to mitigate problems that might arise from one individual managing the entire account. However, with appropriate supervision, challenges to internal controls may be overcome.

There are many other areas where work functions can be linked, with cross-training of staff. As examples:

- A staff member who manages account follow-up can also work denials, or
- A staff member who conducts registration can also address front-end claim edits.

These staffing models permit staff to have a full scope of work function and be held accountable for their performance.

CREATE A PROCESS-DEPENDENT REVENUE CYCLE

Take steps to ensure your revenue cycle is process-dependent rather than people-dependent. Crosstrain staff to ensure that no key process simply waits, regardless of the circumstances.

All too often we have visited medical practices and have found that important work is simply waiting for a staff member to a) find time to focus on the task, b) return from leave, or c) be hired to fill a staff vacancy. The problem with this staffing model is that process steps in the revenue cycle are highly interconnected and revenue can fluctuate at dangerous levels if even one of the processes is significantly delayed.

As an example, let's suppose that the staff member assigned to work claim edits is on leave for two weeks and no one has been delegated this work in her absence. Claim edits are created when the clearinghouse reviews a claim that is queued for submission to a payer, and the system determines an error. The clearinghouse moves the claim(s) into an edit work queue, and flags the error. The claim(s) remains in this queue, awaiting correction until the employee returns from leave. When the staff member does return to the office she is facing a bolus of work, creating even further delays in correcting the claim edits for claim submission — and importantly, delaying revenue to the practice.

For every function in the business office, train a minimum of two staff members to perform the task. Because every revenue cycle process is inter-related, this model not only ensures that work is covered, but it also adds value to staff members as they increase understanding of how each function works.

> EMPHASIZE PROCESS DEPENDENCY. FOR EVERY BUSINESS OFFICE FUNCTION, TRAIN A MINIMUM OF TWO STAFF MEMBERS TO PERFORM THE TASK.

EVALUATE NEW REVENUE CYCLE ROLES

Determine if new roles and responsibilities need to be delegated to staff in support of your revenue cycle. As examples:

- *Reimbursement analysis:* Designated staff to review financial data to determine contract compliance and develop business intelligence to optimize reimbursement.

- *Systems support:* Information technology employees or vendors to create pre-adjudication claim edits, update software modules, interface technologies, and analyze data in multiple formats.

- *Training and quality assurance:* Training staff to orient and provide continuing education to employees and audit work for quality.

Evaluate your current staffing model to determine if your medical practice would benefit from heightened attention to these and other areas.

CONDUCT STAFF COMPETENCY ASSESSMENTS

Conduct formal competency assessments before staff utilize the practice management system with live data. An untrained employee reconciling the electronic remittance advices (ERAs) to the system, for example, can wreak havoc on a system by inadvertently creating credit balances, selecting improper adjustment codes and failing to flag invoices for appeal. Conduct periodic competency assessment for current employees as well. Changes in regulations related to the revenue cycle, updates to the practice management system, and revisions in payer requirements underscore the need to provide ongoing competency evaluations.

Additional staffing innovations and work process redesign for the business office can be found in our book: *The Physician Billing Process: Navigating Potholes on the Road to Getting Paid.*[6]

STAFFING FOR CONSUMER-DIRECTED HEALTH PLANS

Patients are paying more and more out of pocket for their care as part of an intentional cost-share strategy between payers (and/or employers) and patients. Consumer-directed healthcare plans typically require higher financial levels of copayment, co-insurance, and deductible to be paid by patients. These plans commonly involve a high deductible, which must be met by the patient prior to the insurer paying for services.

What this means for the medical practice is that patients are more financially engaged in their care and more of the medical practice's revenue stream is derived from patients, not insurers. Although the patient may have private insurance, if he or she has a $5,000 deductible plan, much of the patient's cost of care within a given year may be the patient's full responsibility (paid up to the practice-payer contract allowable level). This is challenging for medical practices that typically have tight margins and must now attempt to collect more than a small copayment from patients at the point of care.

Collecting from patients after services are performed is more difficult and costlier than making attempts to collect from patients when they are in the medical practice. Consequently, evaluate changes to the staffing model and the work processes allocated to staff.

We recommend that staff be assigned to conduct the work of patient financial clearance prior to the patient being seen. This includes:

- Insurance verification
- Benefits eligibility
- Determining patient financial responsibility (including prior account balance identification)
- Price estimation

See Chapter 6, Staffing the Front Office for a detailed discussion.

If the decision is made not to conduct patient financial clearance, the work is still being performed, it is just a different kind of work at a higher cost. In this example, if patient financial clearance is not performed to ensure that a clean claim is submitted to the payer, business office staff need to be deployed to appeal a claim that may have been denied due to incorrect or inaccurate insurance coverage or benefits, or other similar reasons.

This discussion is consistent with one of the themes of this book: pulling work into the practice. It is simply a different timing and approach to the work and, consequently, a different staffing deployment model to ensure the work is done earlier in the process (prior to the service being performed), rather than later (after the claim has been submitted, adjudicated, and denied).

Examples of the work required for patient financial clearance in markets where consumer-directed healthcare plans are prevalent are listed in Exhibit 8.2. The work of patient financial clearance is typically managed by front office staff; however, some medical practices will involve business office staff. High-performing practices often maintain a staff member(s) dedicated to this function. The various staffing strategies in use today to conduct patient financial clearance functions are described in Chapter 6, Staffing the Front Office.

Exhibit 8.2 Patient Financial Clearance Work Functions

Patient Financial Clearance

- Insurance verification
- Benefits eligibility
  - Authorization
  - Waivers
- Financial responsibility
  - Account balance
  - Copayment level
  - Co-insurance, deductible
  - Credit worthiness
  - Financial risk assessment
  - Price estimation

Staffing for Value-Based Reimbursement

Healthcare reimbursement models are also changing. As more and more payers elect to pay differentially based on performance or value, the work of staff in the medical practice must change. Staff serve an important role in demonstrating performance and outcomes consistent with quality and cost targets and/or demonstrating performance that is of high value, particularly if the medical practice is at financial risk for payment related to these aspects of a payer contract.

> If your practice participates in risk-based reimbursement, redesign your staffing model to include new roles, infrastructure and coding resources.

New Roles

Value-based reimbursement creates new requirements for staff members in a medical practice. Beyond clinical staff involvement in documenting quality and value, the business office of today is faced with the daunting task of managing mixed model reimbursement — fee-for-service plus many other arrangements, to include bundled payments, pay-for-performance, per member per month models, accountable care distributions, and others.

Consider expanding the business office staffing model to include business intelligence, coding, and mixed model reimbursement management to ensure your practice is competitive.

Business Intelligence

The required business intelligence for value-based reimbursement also changes the staffing pattern in a medical practice. Determine if one or more of the following staffing changes are warranted for your medical practice.

Technology

Hire new staff or task existing staff with enhancing the technology proficiency of the practice, to include clinical information systems and data and decision support analysis.

- Staff must become more sophisticated due to the need to document, monitor and report data, to include the use of advanced imaging, generic medications, and patient-specific interventions, as well as information about the health of the patient population or a care episode for bundled payments, and

- The practice is often required to report on a variety of quality measures, thus necessitating a staff member(s) to ensure that the data are entered in such a way to permit abstraction and reporting.

Patient Population Management

Hire or designate a registered nurse(s) (or other appropriately licensed staff) for population health management, to include program development and infrastructure to manage the practice's overall patient population or a cohort of patients in accordance with contractual requirements, such as an at-risk agreement for quality and costs. This involves:

- Determining completeness of care pursuant to established clinical protocols,

- Engaging physicians, advanced practice providers, and the overall care team in care delivery, and

- Monitoring quality outcomes and measures, and other important data as part of the mission of the practice as a medical home and/or the contractual obligation with the payer.

PERFORMANCE METRICS AND MONITORING

Identify or otherwise assign staff to assist practice stakeholders in determining performance targets and metrics and ensuring the provision of evidence-based patient care, to include:

- Creating operational definitions of the metrics,

- Implementing workflow to accommodate measures,

- Educating physicians, advanced practice providers, and other members of the care team regarding the measures, and

- Coaching, educating, and engaging patients in their health and wellness.

DATA ANALYTICS AND REPORTING

Identify or otherwise assign staff to conduct data analytics and reporting, to include:

- Providing physicians, advanced practice providers and other care team members with their performance outcomes to learn their progress toward established targets and goals, and

- Verifying the accuracy of payer reporting of your practice's success on performance metrics which involves sophisticated knowledge and skill, as well as comprehension regarding changing payer reporting requirements.

CODING

To successfully participate in value-based reimbursement, create a dedicated coding staff (either in-house, via vendor or in combination) to perform, educate and/or audit for appropriate procedure and diagnosis coding. Diagnosis coding must receive heightened attention.

- Diagnosis codes, which have historically been of importance, but not vital to the level of reimbursement, become a critical factor in value-based reimbursement, and

- Diagnosis codes provide the framework for the medical necessity of services rendered, as well as define the acuity of the patient.

If the practice is at-risk for quality and/or cost, these elements are vital to appropriate reimbursement. Consequently, in a value-based environment, the role and importance of coders is elevated, and their requisite knowledge is in high demand.

MIXED MODEL REIMBURSEMENT MANAGEMENT

Consider skills expansion to effectively manage mixed model reimbursement where revenue is derived from multiple sources beyond fee-for-service reimbursement. New models of reimbursement may include:

- *Bundled payments.* A single payment provided for an episode of care, typically provided prospectively.

- *Care management.* A periodic payment (commonly monthly) for handling a cohort of patients.

- *Shared incentives.* An established goal related to quality, cost and/or other factors, with payments shared among the parties if achieved.

Administering a mixed-model revenue cycle requires enhanced skills training to ensure that each segment of the revenue stream is well-managed, to include patient tracking and revenue and expense monitoring.

As we describe, medical practices that participate in risk-based arrangements must create staffing models that ensure that the medical practice performs the appropriate work and, importantly, achieves the expected clinical and patient outcomes of that work, in addition to ensuring financial remuneration consistent with contract terms.

KEY QUESTIONS TO ADDRESS

As you analyze the staffing model for your business office, ask and answer the following key questions.

- Is the staff performing at levels that vary from the expected range? Why? There may be valid reasons a business office appears to be overstaffed. If, for example, one of your primary payers is Workers' Compensation, which commonly requires medical documentation to be submitted periodically for payment consideration, your practice may require more staffing resources for billing and collection processes.

- Is the business office leveraging technology to its fullest extent or are staff performing manual tasks that could be automated?

- Is there opportunity to improve the performance of the business office? Do you have the right staff performing the right activities?

- How many functions have been delegated to the staff? Is this multitasking impacting the efficiency of staff in performing any single work function?

- Are the work processes to which the staff adhere encumbered or streamlined?

- Can you explore how other medical practices perform this function so you can learn new ways to improve these processes?

- Does the EHR system, practice management system, and clearinghouse offer the functionality needed to perform at optimal levels? Are you using these management information systems appropriately?

- Do you deploy other technology available in the industry to leverage your human resources?

- Are you effectively organizing and prioritizing work?

- Have you provided the resources for your staff members to be successful in their work?

Summary

In this chapter, we present important tools to help you build your staffing model, including the key work functions for staff involved in billing and collection functions and the expected workload ranges of the staff. Innovative staffing models for billing and collection activity include a decided emphasis on front-end billing and enhanced sophistication to manage value-based reimbursement.

Endnotes

1 MGMA DataDive for Cost and Revenue. All rights reserved. Reprinted with permission.

2 Walker Keegan, Deborah and Elizabeth W. Woodcock. 2016. The Physician Billing Process: Navigating Potholes on the Road to Getting Paid. Englewood, Colo.: Medical Group Management Association.

3 Ibid.

4 Ibid.

5 Woodcock, Elizabeth W. 2007. "Total account ownership: A new model for streamlining your business office staff." MGMA Connexion. 7(1):28–33.

6 Walker Keegan, Deborah and Elizabeth W. Woodcock. 2016. The Physician Billing Process: Navigating Potholes on the Road to Getting Paid. Eglewood, Colo.: Medical Group Management Association.

CHAPTER 9

STAFFING FOR VALUE-BASED CARE

M edical practices are turning their attention to new value-based care delivery models to meet the promise of high quality and low cost amid the overall landscape of healthcare reform. Importantly, innovative delivery models are emerging that offer added personalized value to patients, to include partnering with patients as they live their lives — ensuring access to information and care when and where they need it. The overall goal is to meet patient demand by delivering an experience that offers optimal value to the patients served.

The work associated with value-based care cannot simply be piled higher and higher on the current staff of a medical practice. Instead, new staffing models, changing roles and responsibilities, and potentially additional staff are needed to ensure success.

In this chapter, we:

- Share an example of value-based care
- Define value-based care delivery models
- Discuss staffing strategies for value-based care
- Discuss new staffing roles for a value-based care team
- Provide key questions to address in the transition to value-based care

EXAMPLE OF VALUE-BASED CARE

From the patient's point of view, most of the steps in the traditional patient flow process are not value-added. Calling the practice to schedule an appointment (and often playing telephone tag), waiting for the appointment, checking in at the front office, and again queuing at the check-out station after the visit are sequential steps that most patients simply endure. The only value-added portion of the visit from the perspective of the patient is receiving a diagnosis and treatment plan.

What if we redesigned the patient flow process to focus on value from the patient's perspective? Picture a new model:

- The patient submits a secure message to her care team to describe a health issue,

- The physician orders a test that same day and the patient is notified of the order and instructions via the portal,

- The patient utilizes a mobile health device that transmits the test data to the ordering physician via secure electronic means,

- The results of the test are securely, electronically transmitted to the patient with next step recommendations. In this example, the patient's care team notifies the patient that an ultrasound is recommended, with the patient asking pertinent questions via the portal. The care team member sends the order to the imaging center,

- The imaging center sends a secure, electronic link for the patient to self-schedule her appointment with instructions that she should be seen in the next 48 hours for the test,

- The patient travels to the imaging center for her ultrasound, and

- The results of the ultrasound are transmitted to the ordering physician and the patient the same day via secure, electronic communication, with the patient offered a video visit to discuss the findings and next steps.

In a traditional medical practice, this episode of care with the patient involves multiple face-to-face visits and significant delays. In a practice focused on the delivery of value-based care, prompt access is built into the delivery system, with efforts expended to reduce even this limited number of process steps. Importantly, the staffing model of this medical practice will differ dramatically from the traditional medical practice.

VALUE-BASED CARE DELIVERY MODELS

Three value-based care delivery models will now be discussed:

1. high-performing primary care,

2. primary care medical home, and

3. value-based specialty care.

HIGH-PERFORMING PRIMARY CARE

Many primary care practices are serving their patients in new ways to provide personalized care to patients. These practices are often referred to as advanced or high-performing primary care models. In these models:

- A care team works to ensure that patients are highly engaged and active in their care,

- Patients have access to care 24/7 and a team of clinicians and staff, to include care and case managers, health and wellness coaches, behavioral health specialists, pharmacists, social workers, nurses, and support staff, are assembled to work with patients to help them maintain their health and wellness and manage transitions of care, and

- In turn, patients are encouraged to use expanded access methods to engage with their care team beyond the face-to-face, episodic visit of the traditional medical practice and become active in self-care.

Staffing strategies in these models are different from the traditional staffing model of a primary care practice in the following ways:

- Nursing staff are assigned to manage inbound calls and secure messages using a real-time, one-touch strategy,

- Clinical support staff prepare for the visit by accessing EHR system-based alerts, registries and clinical decision support tools to determine recommended and outstanding services required for the patient,

- The status of the patient is routinely reviewed by the care team, with next steps actively managed and communicated to the patient,

- The patient population is actively managed with a focus on preventive and recommended care, often by a staff member dedicated to panel management, and

- Transitions of care between physicians, such as primary care to specialty care, as well as in and out of facilities, such as hospital discharge, are coordinated by staff assigned to this function.

In short, rather than having patients access care in the office or emergency department only when an acute need arises, the primary care practice deploys a care team to partner with its patients throughout their journey to health and wellness.

Primary Care Medical Home

Some primary care practices have pursued designation as patient-centered medical homes. In a medical home model, patients are assigned to a primary care physician; however, the patient benefits from an entire care team supporting the delivery of care. The care team varies in composition based on the specialty of the practice, the preferences of the practice's owners, the needs of the patients, as well as the availability of personnel. The team, which often includes an advanced practice provider, nurse(s) and/or medical assistant(s), may also encompass a health coach, panel manager, behavioral health counselor, social worker, dietician, nutritionist, or one of many other supporting clinicians. The care team may serve just one physician, or be split among several. Regardless of the composition of the care team, the intent of this model is to provide access, communication, and coordination to assist patients in maintaining health and wellness. Given these goals, a new staffing deployment model is required.

Staff are assigned roles and responsibilities that:

- Facilitate proactive outreach and assistance to patients to support them in receiving recommended, preventive care, as well as to minimize more costly care, such as that provided in an emergency department, and

- Coordinate care, not only with specialists and during the transitions of care, but also with caregivers, to include spouses, guardians, family members and others who provide support to the patient.

The model varies greatly between practices, but it is a break from the past in its proactive service to patients. This contrasts with a traditional practice that primarily manages patients on an episodic basis when acute issues arise.

> IN A MEDICAL HOME MODEL, PATIENTS ARE ASSIGNED TO A PRIMARY
> CARE PHYSICIAN, AND THE PHYSICIAN AND CARE TEAM PROVIDE
> ACCESS AND OUTREACH TO PATIENTS ON A 24/7 BASIS.

A medical home is a practice that caters to the patient in a unique way. The key components of the medical home include the following:

- *Personal physician:* A personal physician is assigned to each patient and is the team leader for a support staff who are collectively responsive to the patient and patient's family or caregiver for comprehensive care.

- *Access to care:* Multiple access channels are available to the patient to meet his or her healthcare needs, with each channel requiring the assignment of staff resources. These include:

  - Expanded access to face-to-face visits with the personal physician and team members,

  - 24/7 access to the care team, and

  - Remote, non-patient-facing care involving the telephone, secure electronic messages, and other mobile health and telemedicine exchanges with patients and caregivers.

- *Transitions of care:* The team members coordinate transitions of care and ensure the full gamut of the patient's health needs are met. Managing transitions of care refers to addressing each of the needs of patients to ensure a well-coordinated and seamless transition as patients move from primary to specialty care, as well as from the hospital to skilled nursing facility and hospital to home. Moreover, the practice maintains a workflow and staffing resources to have knowledge of and manage these transitions, a process that was largely up to the patient and his or her family in years past.

- *Coordination of care:* In a practice that is a medical home, the care team coordinates care for the patient. The coordination of care is facilitated by EHR systems, health information exchanges, registries, telemedicine, and other modalities to ensure timely and appropriate care for the patient.

- *Focus on value:* Quality and safety are paramount in a medical home model:

  ◉ Evidence-based, clinical decision support tools are systematically deployed,

  ◉ Patients are involved in shared decision-making with their physician,

  ◉ Patients are active in self-management, with tools and resources provided to enable patient engagement, and

  ◉ Quality and cost measures often extend beyond the level of a unique patient to that of a patient population.

COORDINATION OF CARE IS FACILITATED BY EHR SYSTEMS, HEALTH INFORMATION EXCHANGES, REGISTRIES, TELEMEDICINE, AND OTHER MODALITIES TO ENSURE TIMELY AND APPROPRIATE CARE FOR THE PATIENT, REQUIRING STAFFING RESOURCES AND NEW WORKFLOW DESIGNS.

This approach to care requires a financial model distinct from traditional fee-for-service reimbursement. Insurers may offer fee-for-service plus incentive or bonus payments, care or case management fees, bundled payments, per member per month payments and/or shared savings distributions based on quality and cost indicators.

VALUE-BASED SPECIALTY CARE

The delivery of value-based care is not limited to primary care. Specialty practices can also be medical homes for patients, providing collaborative care with patients and their families/caregivers. These specialty medical homes have many of the same features as a primary care medical home; care team members are deployed to ensure access and transitions of care. Care coordination is provided to patients.

In addition, many specialty practices are launching telemedicine programs. As examples:

- A neurologist engaged in a telestroke program can provide immediate access for an emergency medicine physician to consult with him or her via video-conference.

- For non-emergent situations that necessitate a consultation with a cardiologist, rather than the patients traveling to a cardiologist, patients can remain in their home, in their primary care physician's office — or in fact, anywhere where the technology resides.

- A psychiatrist can meet face-to-face with a new patient on the first visit, with follow-up at more frequent intervals via video-conferencing.

Telemedicine expands patient access while minimizing staffing and facility resources. As an example, a telemedicine visit eliminates the need for patient check-in, patient check-out and patient-facing visit support; and the required space is limited to the telemedicine equipment.

STAFFING STRATEGIES FOR VALUE-BASED CARE

Regardless of the specific model, as medical practices embrace value-based care, new staffing models to align with new roles and new services are needed.

Value-based care requires a heightened involvement of clinical support staff, including registered nurses (RNs), licensed practical nurses (LPNs), and medical assistants (MAs). Other healthcare professionals — behavioral health specialists, pharmacists, and so forth — supplement the team. In addition, patients are more actively engaged in their care, thus becoming extensions of the care team themselves. Patients use mobile health devices to track key biometric indicators, actively compile and maintain their own health information, and prioritize compliance with recommended and preventive care. The medical practice must allocate resources to support patients in self-care. Finally, value-based care practices are designed to support the patient population of the practice, not just individual patients who express acute needs. This, too, requires new staffing roles and work delegation.

Take the following steps to align your staffing model with value-based care.

CLINICAL ENGAGEMENT IN VALUE PROPOSITION

Determine the value metrics to be reported by your practice and align staff accordingly. This may include new work delegation to clinical support staff, identifying staff to provide oversight of clinical protocols, assigning staff to data capture and reporting, and other similar work functions.

Physicians and clinical staff must not only understand the value proposition (to include appropriateness of care, quality, and costs), but also change their workflow — and often work delegation to staff — to ensure that the practice can successfully demonstrate value. As an example, there is a need to document, monitor, and report data related to advanced imaging, generic medications, and patient-specific interventions.

PATIENT ACCESS CHANNELS

Determine your current — and planned future — patient access channels and reengineer your staffing model. This work cannot simply be piled higher on the work of staff already fully deployed in medical practice. Instead, a well-designed staffing model that ensures knowledgeable staff deployed to each of your patient access channels is warranted.

Today's delivery systems provide expanded patient access channels beyond the traditional face-to-face visit. Patient access channels now include:

- Secure electronic messaging between the patient and the care team,
- Clinical consultation and advice with nurses and/or providers,
- 24/7 management of the patient facilitated by access to electronic health records from anywhere,
- Remote care, involving e-visits via telephone, video, and other media, and telediagnostics,
- Portal access to referral management, self-scheduling, test results reporting, prescription management, education, electronic statements, and bill pay,
- Patient navigation to assist with patient access and care management,
- Group visits, and
- Home care.

VALUE-ADDED SERVICES

As your practice embraces new modalities designed to better meet patient needs for high quality, low cost care, change your staffing deployment model and work assignment of staff to manage new roles and responsibilities. The following value-added services require aligned staffing strategies:

- Outreach care management,
- Health and wellness coaching,
- Coordination and support through transitions of care,
- Self-directed care,
- Support groups,
- Individualized care, and
- Population health and panel management.

These work functions are in addition to those needed to provide the infrastructure and support for the patient-facing encounter with the provider.

> EXPANDED PATIENT ACCESS CHANNELS AND NEW VALUE-ADDED SERVICES REQUIRE CHANGES TO THE STAFFING MODEL OF A MEDICAL PRACTICE.

PATIENT ACTIVATION AND ENGAGEMENT

Assign staff to manage new technologies to engage patients in maintaining or improving their health and wellness. Determine the role of your staff in each of the following technologies:

- Medical devices,
- Wearable technologies and biosensors,
- Patient portals,
- Patient health records,
- Patient logs and journals,
- Electronic medication summaries,

- After-visit summaries,
- Online wellness plans,
- Self-testing and self-management,
- Support groups, and
- Online tools, videos, and graphs.

Formally assign staff to manage the currency of the technology, monitor and oversee the information shared with patients, respond to patients' inquiries and contributions to their records, and other similar work.

A summary of new roles and responsibilities for value-based care is outlined in Exhibit 9.1.

EXHIBIT 9.1 NEW VALUE-BASED CARE ROLES

Patient Access	Care Coordination	Population Health
- Patient navigation - Secure messaging - Telemedicine - Telediagnostics - Group visits - Home visits	- Individual care planning - Registry maintenance - Care management - Motivational interviewing - Health coaching - Device tracking - Transition management	- Panel management - Patient engagement - Value demonstration - Data analysis

DETERMINE THE ROLE OF YOUR STAFF IN PATIENT ACTIVATION, TO INCLUDE DEFINING POLICIES AND PROCEDURES AND PROVIDING EDUCATION AND TRAINING TO MANAGE MULTIPLE TECHNOLOGIES.

THE VALUE-BASED CARE TEAM

The care team in a patient-centered practice is focused on delivering value to patients, family, and caregivers. These practices typically have a higher volume of advanced practice providers and clinical support staff than a traditional practice. Based on MGMA data, physician-owned multispecialty groups that are designated as patient-centered medical homes report 25.71% more nonphysician providers and 10.16% more clinical staff on a per FTE physician basis, as compared to their counterparts.[1]

Importantly, the number and skill mix of staff vary based on how the practice is defined and the services that are provided. If a practice anticipates patients' needs by providing information and outreach to patients, a different staffing model will be required from one that focuses on treating patients in the office for face-to-face visits based on appointments they request. In most of the high-performing models, higher levels of clinical support are required to manage the various access channels for patients and to conduct the care management and outreach functions typical of these delivery systems.

The following caregivers and support staff are typically found in a value-based care model or the patient is directly connected to one of these caregivers as appropriate.

PHYSICIANS

The physician in a patient-centered model is most commonly a primary care physician, specializing in internal medicine, family practice, geriatrics, or pediatrics. The physician, however, does not necessarily need to be a primary care physician. He or she must assume a whole-person orientation toward the patient. For example, an obstetrician/gynecologist, infectious disease physician, or non-invasive cardiologist could likely qualify if he or she assumes all the internal medicine services of the patient. The physician assumes a leadership role within the care team, yet the focus is on all aspects of serving the patient and his or her family and caregivers.

ADVANCED PRACTICE PROVIDERS

One or more advanced practice providers, such as a physician assistant or nurse practitioner, may be a member of the care team. Their role varies based on the work assigned as well as their scope of practice, however, these clinicians provide a vital role in the care team. They may serve in a role to support the physician in delivering care, or they may be the featured clinician whom patients may choose as their primary clinician.

CLINICAL SUPPORT STAFF

The work of ensuring that the patient's care and treatment are consistent with evidence-based guidelines and established targets and goals rests with the physician and clinical support staff, necessitating a change to staffing work scope and effort. As examples:

- Clinical protocols and evidence-based guidelines guide care delivery and patient outcomes are documented and reported.

- Registries and electronic health record systems assist in identifying preventive, recommended and outstanding clinical services required of patients.

- Clinical staff are highly involved in visit preparation, patient outreach, patient education, and patient self-management to demonstrate patient compliance, intervention, and outcomes.

The care team typically includes a registered or licensed practical nurse(s) who manages communication from patients. Communication may be received via an inbound telephone call or a secure, electronic message. These communications may require triage and/or advice. In some practices, the nurse may filter all messages — or respond to the communication upon physician review and approval. This nurse may also contact patients regarding their test results, by telephone or secure electronic means.

One or more of the nurses on the care team typically receives and responds to inbound telephone calls from patients. These staff also typically manage secure, electronic messages sent by patients. The volume of work expected is 65 to 85 calls per day, or eight to 12 per hour, which is five to eight minutes per inquiry (assuming a seven-hour productive day) (see Chapter 4, Staff Productivity for additional workload measures). The nurses may reside in the medical practice or alternatively, telecommute from a remote location with access to the EHR system.

> THE ROLE OF CLINICAL SUPPORT STAFF HAS EXPANDED WITH VALUE-BASED CARE. THEY MUST BECOME HIGHLY INVOLVED IN VISIT PREPARATION, PATIENT OUTREACH, PATIENT EDUCATION, AND PATIENT SELF-MANAGEMENT.

CARE MANAGERS

Care managers are typically registered or licensed nurses who manage a designated panel of patients in accordance with contractual requirements, such as an at-risk agreement for quality and costs, or the practice's overall patient population. They may also be referred to as panel managers. Both the responsibilities of the role, as well as the patients served vary by practice.

In many practices, care managers:

- Determine completeness of care pursuant to established clinical protocols,

- Engage physicians, advanced practice providers, and the overall team in care delivery,

- Monitor quality outcomes and measures,

- Communicate with the patient, family, and/or caregiver to ensure that the patient is complying with the plan of care, and

- Support the patient in self-management, coordinating the patient's care with specialists, and providing guidance for medications and other between-visit care.

Using a registry or other database tool as a resource, the care manager may contact the patient one or more times per month to converse with the patient about his or her plan of care, as well as provide support and education, responding to any questions from the patient, family member or caregiver. The role is purposefully loosely defined, primarily because every patient has different needs.

The practice may assign the care manager to assist patients who are identified as high risk, based on their condition or disease state. Assignments may also be made based on multiple chronic care conditions, historical patterns of admissions and emergency department utilization, and/or those who need outreach support.

Depending on the complexity of the assigned patient cohort, and the extent of the care manager's role, the volume of assigned patients may vary from a small group — 10 to 50 patients — to an entire panel of 1,000-plus patients. The frequency of interaction with assigned patients will also often vary based on acuity. As an example, a low acuity patient may receive one outreach communication monthly, while a patient with high acuity who is more complex may receive two or more communications each week. To measure productivity, it's important to determine how many patients will be served by this role, the patient complexity, and the work scope delegated. The higher the acuity and more complex the patients are, the lower the number of patients served.

Transition Managers

A transition manager is typically a nurse or other qualified staff who is focused on managing transitions of care. As examples:

- A primary care patient may need to see a specialist. The transition manager provides the patient's information to the specialist and coordinates records flow, referrals, and scheduling.

- A patient is discharged from the hospital. The transition manager is involved in the hospital discharge and manages the patient's transfer from hospital to home care (or other setting), providing a seamless transition.

This may be a distinct role or the duties may be assumed by the care manager, as discussed above.

Nurse Navigators

We discuss nurse navigators in Chapter 7, Staffing the Encounter. There is no standard role for a nurse navigator. They can be assigned to manage transitions of care, assist new patients with access and visit itineraries and/or ensure a consistent point of contact for complex patients with clinical issues.

Health and Wellness Coaches

The deployment of a health and wellness coach depends on the coach's licensure and skill level, as well as the type of coaching performed. For example, a wellness coach may reach out to patients who have adopted a weight loss program to ensure they are on track. A health coach may proactively communicate with patients who are on certain medications, ensuring they are taking them as prescribed and reviewing any side effects they are having. With today's technology, health and wellness coaches are increasingly involved in reminders to patients, such as sending text messages to patients to remind them of their blood pressure checks, glucose monitoring, and other self-care aids. This coaching function may be a distinct role, a coach with whom the practice contracts, or it may be the responsibility of the care manager as part of his or her duties.

The workload for health coaches depends on the type of coaching they provide. Caseloads are highly variable based on type and approach. A health coach may be on the telephone, secure messaging, or other communication channel upwards of six hours per day, with many of them teleworking rather than residing in the medical practice.

CLINICAL PHARMACISTS

Medications represent a vital part of patients' care plans. Historically, patients have been sent away from practices with a directive to head to their pharmacy to pick up one or more medications. Adherence to the medication, as well as taking the prescribed dosage and duration, have been the patient's responsibility. Awareness regarding the importance of managing this critical aspect of the plan of care has led to practices employing, contracting, or working closely with pharmacists.

Like other support roles, the responsibilities vary by practice. In many, however, a clinical pharmacist is assigned to patients to review medication management, side effects, and refill and renewal activity. The pharmacist may also be involved in anticoagulation management and other similar long-term medication management for the patient. The pharmacist often serves patients in concert with physician encounters, but may also have his or her own schedule to work with patients in the office.

Regardless of the details of the position, the pharmacist is a valuable member of the care team, helping patients manage their medications and thereby improving the quality of care for patients taking multiple medications, suffering multiple chronic care conditions, or those who have medication allergies or sensitivities.

BEHAVIORAL HEALTH SPECIALISTS

Historically, medical practices focused exclusively on patients' medical needs, however, patients' health depends on their behavioral and emotional needs as well. Patients also may need assistance with personal challenges that may incorporate family life, housing, food, addictions, employment, and/or finances. If the patient's whole-person is not treated, he or she will not be healthy. Thus, this is a crucial role of the care team.

The practice may employ a behavioral health specialist, or contract or refer patients to one. Often trained as licensed psychologists, professional counselors or social workers, the specialist focuses on patients in the office, as well as communicates with patients between face-to-face encounters. He or she may also make home visits. A behavior health specialist often works in close collaboration with a psychiatrist. This role has become commonplace in medical homes, particularly based on reimbursement opportunities that cover many of these services.

DATA MANAGERS/ANALYSTS

Success depends on the ability of the practice to demonstrate value. This requires patient identification, prioritization of resources, performance monitoring, and reporting of quality and cost indices. The ability to query and report on data is vital to the efficiency and effectiveness of a value-based practice. Thus, dedicated resources for information technology — whether they be from an employee or a contractual relationship — is a requirement, as is business intelligence expertise.

FRONT OFFICE SUPPORT STAFF

Front office support staff play important roles in value-based practices. We discuss these roles in Chapter 5, Staffing Communications and Chapter 6, Staffing the Front Office. Building the front office staff model based on the expected productivity staff workload ranges associated with each work function recognizes both the work function and the quantity of work performed by these team members.

DEPLOYMENT OF THE VALUE-BASED CARE TEAM

Exhibit 9.2 depicts a value-based care team model deployed to optimize patient access, extend the reach of clinicians and provide personal, value-based care. It is an example of staff assigned to newer roles as part of a redesigned delivery system.

As depicted in this model, a total of 85 patients received care by the care team during this half-day session. Of these, only one-third of the patients were seen in a traditional face-to-face visit.[2] This expanded patient access involves clinical support staff performing nurse visits, triaging inbound clinical calls, responding to secure messaging, conducting care management, and performing patient navigation.

EXHIBIT 9.2 VALUE-BASED CARE TEAM

Time	MD/DO	APP	NURSE	TRIAGE	SECURE MESSAGE	CARE MNGMT	NAVIGATE	HOME VISIT
9:00	Appt	Appt	Appt	2 Calls	2 Notes	Call	New PT	Visit
9:15	Appt	Appt	Open	2 Calls	2 Notes	Call	New PT	
9:30	2 Appts	Same Day Appt	Appt	2 Calls	2 Notes	Call	Hospital Discharge	
10:00	Phone Visit	Same Day Appt	Appt	Call	2 Notes	Call		
10:15	Same Day Appt	Same Day Appt	Appt	2 Calls	2 Notes	Call	Home Care Transition	Visit
10:30	Same Day Appt	Same Day Appt	Open	2 Calls	2 Notes	Call		
10:45	Video Visit	Phone Visit	Appt	2 Calls	2 Notes	Call		
11:00	Same Day Appt	Video Visit	Appt	Call	2 Notes	Call	Transition to SNF	
11:15	Same Day Appt	Same Day Appt	Appt	Call	2 Notes	Call	Hospital Discharge	Visit
11:30	2 Appts	Same Day Appt	Appt	2 Calls	Note	Call		
Total	12	10	8	17	19	10	6	3
Grand Total								85

APPT = Appointment
PT = Patient
SNF = Skilled nursing facility

KEY QUESTIONS TO ADDRESS

The evolution to value-based care does not occur overnight and medical practices are in different stages in their transition. Market-driven timing of value-based capabilities often is the catalyst for change efforts. To help you explore opportunities to transition to value-based care, brainstorm the exercise outlined in Exhibit 9.3 with your leaders and colleagues.

EXHIBIT 9.3 TRANSITION TO VALUE-BASED CARE EXERCISE

Exercise Scenario: Your practice must transition overnight to accepting full risk. That is, instead of being reimbursed via fee-for-service, your practice will receive a flat fee per patient per month to take care of your patients' healthcare needs.

Exercise Questions to Ask and Answer:

1. What changes to patient access will you adopt? Is it reasonable, for example, to expand to 24/7 nurse triage and/or same day visit access? Does it make sense to begin home care visits?

2. What changes to your staffing model are needed? For example, do you have the right staff in the right roles to manage expanded access and service?

3. What changes to patient outreach and engagement will you adopt? For example, what steps should you take to reduce emergency department visits and hospital admissions? What steps will you take to manage chronic care disease that is different from traditional, episodic visits?

4. What changes need to be made with your referring physicians (inbound and outbound)? For example, are you aware of the "value" of the specialists to which you refer? How can you streamline your referral process to permit seamless care for your patients?

Via visualization and brainstorming of these questions, among others, you can begin to explore the required changes that are needed in a new value-based world.

As you develop your practice's value-based care capabilities, consider the following questions in redesigning your staffing model:

- Have you deployed your care team staff to critical value-based care processes?

- What additional education and/or tools does the staff need to effectively demonstrate value-based care?

- Is it time to embrace a new patient care delivery system, with an aligned staffing model that includes value-based components?

- What episodic visits do you currently have that could be better managed by staff conducting care outreach or via telemedicine?

- Have you taken steps to improve patient access via multiple access channels — and have you appropriately staffed those channels?

- What is the staff's role in helping patients maintain their health and focus on wellness?

- Have you designated staff roles for population health — to include new service offerings and business intelligence?

SUMMARY

In this chapter, we describe value-based care delivery systems and the roles care team members play when assuming a whole-person patient orientation. We also describe new patient access channels and services, requiring new roles and responsibilities of the care team. Adopting value-based care directly impacts not only your patients, but also the staffing roles and staffing deployment model of a medical practice.

ENDNOTES

1 Custom analysis of the Medical Group Management Association 2016 Cost Survey database. Copyright 2017 MGMA. Staffing per FTE Physician in Physician Owned Multispecialty Groups by and if the Practice is a Patient-Centered Medical Home. Custom analysis by David N. Gans.

2 In Exhibit 9.2, 29 patients had a traditional face-to-face visit: MD/DO: 10, APP: 8; Nurse: 8; Home Health: 3.

PART 4

How to Optimize Your Staffing Deployment Model

CHAPTER 10

STAFFING
DEPLOYMENT
MODELS

A staffing deployment model outlines the staffing levels and work assignments a medical practice has adopted for key work functions. The model identifies who is to perform the work and how work is to be performed. Staffing models are unique to a medical practice; rarely are too entirely identical.

In this chapter, we:

- Define staffing deployment models

- Learn to analyze a staffing deployment model

- Describe the challenges of traditional staffing models

WHAT IS A STAFFING DEPLOYMENT MODEL?

A staffing deployment model is the overall design of your organization from a staffing perspective, to include the roles and responsibilities assigned and delegated to staff. In contrast with the previous chapters in which we discuss staffing for very specific work functions at a micro-level, the staffing deployment model is the macro-level view of how a medical practice organizes its staff and to whom it assigns generalized work functions.

Rarely do two medical practices have the exact same staffing model. The examples in Exhibits 10.1 and 10.2 demonstrate how the models vary. Exhibit 10.1 reflects two separate staffing deployment models for front office work, and Exhibit 10.2 reflects two models for clinical support.

Exhibit 10.1 Front Office Staffing Model

Medical Practice A

Patients check-in and check-out at the front office. Each front office staff member is tasked with:

- Inbound telephone calls
- Secure messages (administrative)
- Patient check-in
- Patient check-out
- Referral management

Medical Practice B

- Call center staff manage inbound telephone calls, secure messages and referrals.
- When patients arrive for their visit they are escorted to an exam room; patients self-check-in via a portable tablet.
- The medical assistant conducts check-out in the exam room.

EXHIBIT 10.2 CLINICAL SUPPORT STAFFING MODEL

Medical Practice A

A 1.00 staff FTE nurse is assigned to each physician. Each nurse performs an expanded work scope that includes:

- Visit preparation
- Patient retrieval, rooming and intake
- Visit support
- Inbound telephone calls (clinical)
- Secure messages (clinical)
- Patient education and discharge

Medical Practice B

- A 1.00 staff FTE nurse is assigned to manage inbound telephone calls and secure electronic messages for four physicians.
- Medical assistants work in teams, focusing on rooming patients in a steady flow and providing visit support.
- A team nurse travels to the exam room to provide patient education as requested by the physician.

As demonstrated by these examples, each of these medical practices has a unique staffing deployment model with a different definition of who is involved in the work function and how that work function is to be executed.

> A STAFFING DEPLOYMENT MODEL IS THE OVERALL DESIGN OF YOUR ORGANIZATION FROM A STAFFING PERSPECTIVE, TO INCLUDE THE ROLES AND RESPONSIBILITIES ASSIGNED AND DELEGATED TO STAFF.

When the work levels and type of work in a practice change, the staffing model must be realigned to meet these realities. As we discuss in the previous chapter, value-based care involves novel patient access channels and new services that must be effectively staffed. Rather than simply hire more employees, medical practices are carefully scrutinizing their staffing models for opportunities to better align the work throughout the practice.

How to Analyze Your Staffing Model

There are two basic steps to analyze staffing deployment. The first step is to array your current model. The second step is to ask and answer a specific set of questions to understand your current design and assess the changes that can be made to improve your model for the future. Each step is described below.

Step 1: Array Your Current Staffing Deployment Model

Formulate a grid of your current staffing model, as the first step in analyzing the deployment of staff. A sample staffing deployment model is arrayed in Exhibit 10.3. The first column describes the work function. The second column describes who is performing each function. The last column is a summary of how that work function is currently performed.

Exhibit 10.3 Staffing Deployment Model

Work Function	Who	How
Telephones	Front office staff manage inbound telephone calls	The telephones ring in the reception area and are managed by the check-in/check-out staff. Staff either manage the call or take a message for the clinical support staff.
Patient check-in	Front office staff manage patient check-in	Check-in staff receive patients, register new patients, verify and update information with established patient, conduct insurance verification, obtain time-of-service payments, and arrive the patient in the EHR system.
Patient check-out	Front office staff manage patient check-out	Check-out staff schedule follow-up visits and ancillary services, manage outbound referrals, and review or confirm charges.
Clinical support	There is a 1-to-1 assignment of a nurse to a physician	The nurse is responsible for clinical telephone calls and secure electronic messages, as well as patient visit support (including clinical intake) for his or her assigned physician.

By arraying the staffing deployment model, we learn significant information about the medical practice. This medical practice combined the staffing roles for both the patient flow and communications processes, as well as remote care, as follows:

- Front office staff multitask to manage telephones and reception functions.

- Clinical staff multitask to manage patient flow for the face-to-face visit, in addition to telephone calls and secure, electronic messages.

Step 2: Ask and Answer Questions

Once you have arrayed your staffing deployment model, ask and answer questions related to the model. The first question to ask is, "Why have you modeled your staff in this specific fashion?" Often, the answer is that the staffing model was never proactively designed in the first place. Instead, over time, the medical practice grew, expanded, or changed; systems were updated and new workflow implemented; and personal requests from physicians, advanced practice providers and staff were accommodated, resulting in the current staffing model which essentially grew up over time. Although there may be benefits from the current staffing model, many medical practices have not proactively constructed their staffing models to be effective in today's environment.

By asking and answering a standard set of questions, you can determine if there are changes that can be made to your model that will be more effective in supporting the delivery of value-based care and ensuring an optimal patient experience.

> OVER TIME, THE MEDICAL PRACTICE GREW, EXPANDED, OR CHANGED, WHILE THE STAFFING MODEL REMAINED UNALTERED AND IS NO LONGER CURRENT.

Ask and answer the following questions to analyze your staffing deployment model:

- **Work quantity.** Is the quantity of work consistent with the staff volume? (We discuss this concept further in Chapter 4, Staff Productivity.)

- **Work efficiency.** Are the staff efficient in the performance of their functions and tasks? Is there downtime? Are staff rushing around throughout the day or is there a systematic, planned, and focused approach to the work?

- **Work quality.** What is the work quality or outcome of the work? For example, what type of claim edits need to be worked due to problematic registration information? How many rings until the telephone is answered? What is the call abandonment rate? What is the lag time to return secure, electronic messages? Are tests tracked from order to completion, and patients notified about results in a timely manner? What areas do patients complain about in the practice? Is there a staffing deficiency that could be the cause of or contributor to those complaints? Is there a better way to staff the work function so that the work quality and quantity are consistent with expected levels?

- **Work backlog.** Is there work that is not being attended to on a regular basis? Is a backlog creating rework, such as patient messages not being attended to, followed by patients initiating repeat messages or telephone calls to inquire about the status?

- **Provider support.** Are physicians and advanced practice providers fully supported in the scope of their work? Is the clinician wasting time looking for the nurse or retrieving his or her own patients, supplies, and materials for the visit?

- **Skill mix.** Are the nurses working at the full scope of licensure? Are they largely devoted to nursing tasks or to administrative functions, such as scheduling? Is a different skill set required for the work?

- **Work scope.** What duties have providers delegated to staff? Are there additional duties that can be assigned to improve provider efficiency and patient access? Have the appropriate functions been delegated to the right level of staff in the medical practice?

- **Work consolidation.** To what extent have specific work functions been centralized or decentralized? Would consolidating certain work functions enhance practice efficiency and improve performance?

- **Care team.** Are the staff contributing to an integrated care team or are they functioning in silos? Can staff be co-located or can collaborative or team-based approaches to work be developed?

- **Economies of scale.** Is the practice taking advantage of economies of scale? Can work functions be linked with other staff or other parts of the medical practice? Are flexible staffing models deployed?

- **Technology.** Can technology be leveraged? For example, can patients perform some tasks themselves, for example, self-schedule, obtain test results via the portal, register via kiosk upon arrival to the practice or via a tablet while in the exam room?

- **Remote care.** Can more care be performed remotely, such as via secure messaging, telephone, or video visits?

- **Staff accountability.** Are staff present to fulfill the obligations of their assigned functions? Are they able to successfully accomplish these responsibilities while fully participating as a team member? Is the workload balanced among staff members and among care teams?

- **Value-based care.** Are staff performing new roles required for value-based care and value-based reimbursement? Are additional employees needed or can work be re-assigned and/or re-delegated?

By arraying your staffing deployment model and asking critical questions, you can begin to understand potential opportunities to improve the infrastructure and support for physicians and patients. You see the potential to change patient access channels and services offered by your care delivery system.

DRAWBACKS OF TRADITIONAL STAFFING MODELS

The traditional staffing deployment model that is depicted in this chapter does not identify separate and distinct staff involved in the patient flow process (the encounter) from that of communications (the telephones and secure, electronic messaging). When a medical practice maintains this type of blended staffing deployment model, we typically observe less productivity and efficiency than in a medical practice with a more advanced staffing model.

Examples of the challenges borne by practices with traditional staffing models include:

- *High multitasking.* The front office staff are unable to be successful while simultaneously attending to telephones and the patients arriving for visits.

- *High claim edits and denials.* There are significant numbers of claim edits and claim denials because the multitasking staff make more mistakes in securing patients' demographic and insurance information.

- *Reduced time-of-service collections.* The amount of money collected at the point of care is lower than expected, due to the hectic pace of the front office and lack of business planning prior to patient visits.

- *Poor customer experience.* The staff are rushed in their telephone interaction with patients, families, and referring physicians, resulting in poor perceptions of service by customers. In addition, patients perceive the frenetic pace in the practice when they present for care, leading to thoughts such as: "how are they taking care of me, when they can't take care of their office?"

- *Inefficient scheduling.* The staff are not able to optimize the scheduling template due to the competing demands for their time, resulting in physician inefficiency and problematic patient access.

- *Failure to clinically prepare for the visit.* There is little or no visit preparation because clinical support staff are required to manage the visit patient flow, fitting telephone and secure, electronic messaging in between encounters, and do not have adequate time to conduct this work.

- *Inefficient physicians.* The physician rarely starts or ends clinic on time. The physician is typically waiting on staff to receive, arrive and room patients because of staffing inefficiencies at both the front office and among clinical support staff.

- *Premature departure from exam rooms.* Physicians leave the exam room to locate their assigned nurse because the nurse is busy with telephone calls and messages, and is not able to anticipate the patients' and physicians' needs for the visit.

BY ARRAYING YOUR STAFFING MODEL AND ASKING KEY QUESTIONS, YOU BEGIN TO UNDERSTAND POTENTIAL OPPORTUNITIES TO IMPROVE THE INFRASTRUCTURE AND SUPPORT FOR YOUR PHYSICIANS AND PATIENTS.

SUMMARY

In this chapter, we discuss the importance of arraying your current staffing deployment model and asking and answering questions to help determine staffing improvement opportunity. The staffing model in many medical practices was not formally designed in the first place; instead, it grew over time. Thus, many medical practices are recognizing the need to redesign their overall model to effectively compete in a value-based world.

CHAPTER 11

TELEWORKING AND FLEXIBLE STAFFING

Many corporations have worked to facilitate work-life balance and attract and retain talent by instituting teleworking. Healthcare as an industry has lagged in this area; however, opportunities are available should a practice elect to transition from a traditional staffing model of full-time staff physically based at the practice site to one that relies on a workforce that features part-time or per-diem employees, staff participating via a contract or a third-party vendor, or employees working remotely.

The ability to create flexible staffing strategies to respond to fluctuating work volumes and staff shortages is a necessity in a medical practice. "The show must go on" is a perfect description of the life of a medical practice. If employees Bob and Sally both call in sick the same day, the medical practice must still figure out how to function, and function effectively. The patient should not be required to accommodate the practice; ideally, the fact that the practice is not fully staffed on any given day should be transparent to the patient.

In this chapter, we describe:

- Teleworkers
- Part-time and per-diem staff
- Contract workers via a third-party vendor
- Staffing to meet fluctuating work volume
- Staffing to optimize facility utilization
- Work segmentation, extension and rotation strategies

TELEWORKERS

Many work functions in a medical practice can be performed remotely. The definition of "remote" may involve the employee's home — or perhaps the practice has set up an office in a different geographical location. Remote employees truly could be anywhere, if their work can be performed based on their access to the tools they need (and the appropriate confidentiality and security of these tools). Often called telecommuters or teleworkers, these employees can be instrumental to the success of the practice, offering benefits for both employees and the medical practice alike.

The benefits for employees include:

- Flexible work schedule,
- Staff empowerment,
- High morale,
- Enhanced loyalty, and
- Potential increase in staff engagement.

The benefits to the medical practice include:

- Increased productivity (typically due to less work distractions as well as the employee working at a high level so they can continue to be permitted teleworker status),
- Ability to attract and retain a greater talent pool,
- Conversion of office space to that which is revenue generating (or alternatively, a reduction of facility size and expense),
- Ability to work through challenges due to inclement weather, and
- Lower levels of absenteeism.

Probably the chief disadvantage of teleworking programs is the limitation it places on flexibility to permit cross-coverage of employees. Managing teleworkers also requires effort on the part of the practice. Workstations must be set up, as well as parameters for home offices (for example, high-speed internet). Most practices that engage in this strategy require employees to work for a certain time in the office, and even after working remotely, may also require periodic face-to-face "touch bases." Of course, productivity and performance are closely monitored.

Advances in technology permit teleworkers to participate in collective forums, such as meetings, while conducting their work remotely. Witness the many buildings and office locations of staff at some of our largest medical practices. They may be next door, down the street or even across town.

> Advances in technology permit teleworkers to participate in collective forums, such as meetings, while conducting their work from home (or from wherever they have the required access to technology).

Work That May be Performed Remotely

The case can be made that if the staff are not involved in face-to-face visits with the patient and do not need to be co-located to perform their job or cover for a colleague, their work can be performed wherever they have access to the technology and tools they need. The types of positions that are suitable for working from a remote site include the following.

- *Call Center.* Answering the telephone does not require operators to be present in the medical practice. A consolidated call center may be situated across town or employees may be provided with home offices to permit them to telework.

- *Nurse triage and advice.* To assist patients with their out-of-office care, nurses working remotely may participate in responding to patients' requests for advice via telephone and secure, electronic messages; triaging patients to the appropriate care based on a discussion of symptoms; and conferring with patients, families, and caregivers regarding questions about their plan of care. Although co-location of nurses and physicians is often viewed as optimal, the fact is that many physicians are not available to the nurse for in-person communication during the day; much of this interaction is already conducted by telephone, through the electronic health record (EHR) system or via secure messaging.

- *Population health management.* Nurses, medical assistants or administrative support staff may function remotely to work with the practice's patients — or a specific cohort of patients — by communicating with patients via telephone and secure, electronic messaging during transitions of care, coordinating care, reminding patients of recommended and preventive care, and chronic disease management. With a list of patients and their pertinent records, care managers contact patients at home during convenient hours for the patient.

- **Health and wellness coaching.** Similarly, health and wellness coaches work from flow sheets on their patients, a registry and/or the EHR system. They contact patients by telephone or secure messaging wherever they have access to the technology and confidentiality for patient interaction.

- **Coding and charge entry.** Operative reports, procedure notes, and other clinical documentation may be scanned, routed, and/or securely accessed by employees trained in procedure and/or diagnosis coding. The employee records the codes in the practice management system, or documents them on the clinical note, which is subsequently accessed by an employee responsible for entering the charges. Charge entry may be performed in a coordinated fashion with the coder(s), or simply based on documentation directly from the providers.

- **Business office.** In addition to coding and charge entry, there are many other functions in the revenue cycle that lend themselves to remote work. These include, but are not limited to, open claims follow-up, credit balance resolution, insurance follow-up, customer service, and patient collections.

- **Transcription.** So long as the staff member has the appropriate technology, transcription may be conducted off-site. In fact, many healthcare organizations outsource this to other countries.

Whether the staff member is physically based in the medical practice, works in a separate building, or operates from home, it is important to identify the tools and oversight that are required for the work functions and to ensure that privacy and security measures are in place to protect patient data.

POPULATION HEALTH MANAGEMENT MAY BE CONDUCTED REMOTELY BY COMMUNICATING WITH PATIENTS VIA TELEPHONE AND SECURE, ELECTRONIC MESSAGING TO MANAGE TRANSITIONS OF CARE, CARE COORDINATION, PREVENTIVE CARE, AND CHRONIC DISEASE MANAGEMENT.

PART-TIME / PER-DIEM STAFF

If your medical practice has high variability in patient encounter volume and/ or inbound communications by day of week and session per day, consider engaging part-time or per-diem staff. Many practices experience boluses of work and full-time employees may not be able to keep up. If they can't, they are constantly playing catch up, morale dips and furthermore, the patient's experience suffers. To avoid the adverse consequences of these work surges, part-time or per-diem staff can be engaged to handle a portion of the work.

There are two distinct strategies: (1) replace full-time staff with part-time or per-diem staff, thereby optimizing staff scheduling flexibility and (2) employ part-time or per-diem staff to augment your full-time staff.

Part-time staff are typically expected to work less hours than their full-time colleagues; they may or may not receive benefits depending on the number of work hours. Per-diem is a separate category from part-time employees. Per-diem staff typically work fewer hours than part-timers and have no benefits. These staff are vetted by the practice and are often called into the practice to work on short notice. Both part-time and per-diem staff may work the same number of hours, however, per-diem staff typically work on a limited basis.

It is often easy to predict the time of the day when work will surge; it may be based on season (for example, winter); day of week (for example, Mondays) or hour of day (for example, 1:00 to 2:00 p.m.). Or, you may wish to extend office hours but recognize your current workforce cannot handle the extra time. Part-time and per-diem employees can supplement the workforce to ensure optimal performance.

A terrific way to review the immediate opportunity for this model is to analyze the overtime paid by your practice. It's not uncommon for overtime to be higher than that which would be possible via a part-time or per-diem solution. Even if overtime is not a problem, part-time and per-diem staff offer an exceptional solution to labor shortages.

> WITH PART-TIME OR PER-DIEM STAFF ON BOARD, THE MEDICAL
> PRACTICE CAN ACHIEVE PRODUCTIVITY GAINS WHILE MEETING
> PATIENT EXPECTATIONS FOR SERVICE IN A WAY THAT IS DIFFICULT
> FOR THE FULL-TIME STAFF MEMBER WHO IS TRYING TO PLAY CATCH-
> UP AT THE END OF A BUSY WEEK.

BENEFITS OF PART-TIME / PER-DIEM STAFF

Benefits of part-time staffing models include the following:

- *Appropriately resourced practice.* Augmenting full-time staff with part-time assistance when there is high work volume (such as on Mondays) benefits both clinicians and patients, fostering a streamlined patient flow process.

- *Sustained productivity.* With part-time assistance during work peaks, the full-time employee is less likely to go home overly stressed, thereby potentially leading to an increase in employee productivity throughout the week. With part-time staff on board, the medical practice can achieve productivity gains while also meeting patient expectations for service in a way that is difficult for the full-time staff member who is trying to play catch-up at the end of a busy week.

- *Consistent work quality.* With part-time assistance during hectic periods the staff can perform their full work scope rather than work at a rushed pace which may lead to work delays or errors.

- *Reduction in overtime accumulation.* With a part-time staff member supplementing the work of full-time staff, the full-time staff may accrue less overtime (or the part-time staff can stay the extended hours).

RECRUITMENT OF PART-TIME / PER-DIEM STAFF

Recruit part-time staff using the tools provided in Chapter 13, Staff Recruitment, Retention, and Talent Management. Many markets have well-trained medical practice professionals in their community who welcome the opportunity to work part time or per diem. Other sources of part-time and per-diem staff are described as follows.

- **Students.** Students with an interest in healthcare, such as nursing students or pre-med students, can be tapped to work in the medical practice on a part-time or per-diem basis. The position of a scribe for a surgeon during clinic, for example, may be filled by a medical student working per-diem. Some work-study programs may reimburse part of the students' wages for this work.

> STUDENT INTERNS ARE ANOTHER SOURCE OF PART-TIME STAFF. THESE STUDENTS OFTEN HAVE A VESTED INTEREST IN PERFORMING WELL AND CAN BE A VALUABLE ADDITION TO THE CARE TEAM.

- **Interns.** Student interns are another source of part-time or per-diem staff. They can be paid or unpaid, depending on the program. These students often have a vested interest in performing well in the practice because this experience can launch them in their career and/or help them to complete their study requirements. Interns can be an exceptional addition to the traditional full-time staff in a medical practice.

- **Internal float pool.** Given the complexity of the medical practice environment, filling in the gaps with part-time and per-diem staff available in the local market is not always possible. Thus, some practices create an internal workforce that can be accessed for staff coverage needs. Often found in large practices, the goal is to create an internal talent pool with workers scheduled to "float" among positions. Unlike the external market, these floaters are trained in the basic management systems — the practice management system, EHR system, and the telephone system. An internal float pool can be expensive, particularly if it's not well managed. Large practices have found success in combining the float pool with a hire-ahead strategy, which means that the floaters (who are already onboarded and trained) are placed in permanent positions as they become available.

The opportunity to have a cadre of per-diem or part-time staff available to the medical practice should be pursued. Particularly if the workers are engaged on a routine basis, many of these staff members have long-standing relationships with the medical practice and are wholeheartedly committed to its success.

CONTRACT WORKERS

Staffing is a challenging issue for practices, as employees are often needed in short order. In addition to the immediacy, these positions often require technical knowledge. Practices often cannot afford the weeks — or even months — to on-board a new hire with the skills, knowledge, and experience needed for the job. Contract workers — available through a staffing agency that focuses on this area of contingency staffing — or via a relationship with a third-party vendor that specializes in a work function needed by the practice (for example, patient collections) — can offer significant value to a practice. These relationships vary by practice, but often feature contractors working during current employees' leave, between staff departures and new hires, and/or when there is increased work volume based on season. The labor may be temporary (often referred to as a temp), or temporary but expected to be filled on a permanent basis (a temp-to-perm). The practice may also choose the contractor option on a long-term basis, as there may be opportunities to more easily replace a staff vacancy, bypass organizational requirements or budgetary constraints related to the number or expense of employees, as well as potentially save staff benefit costs.

Contract workers can prevent challenges emanating from having unfilled positions throughout the practice: telephones ringing without anyone to answer them, patients calling for appointments without anyone to schedule them, physicians needing assistance in the procedure room without anyone to help, or patients' inquiries about statement balances going unanswered. The scenarios are endless, as the work of a practice never stops, even when an employee departs. Using contract workers or developing a relationship with a third-party vendor to fill vacancies by using their employees or services to fill in the gaps, can help practices avoid challenges that hit their bottom lines.

STAFFING TO MEET FLUCTUATING WORK VOLUME

In many medical practices, physicians are not present in the office setting five days per week, eight hours per day. Patient visit volume fluctuates by day of week and session per day. The work of staff members involved in the patient visit is therefore variable, consistent with the visit volume fluctuations.

> WITH FLUCTUATING PATIENT VISIT VOLUME, A STATIC STAFFING MODEL MEANS THAT THE MEDICAL PRACTICE WILL EITHER BE OVERSTAFFED OR UNDERSTAFFED FOR THE WORK.

Many medical practices incur a high staffing cost because they are not actually staffing for the work. In these medical practices, staff are assigned a static schedule, such as 8:00 a.m. to 5:00 p.m., regardless of the volume of work to be performed. If the physician is in surgery, rounding at the hospital, or at meetings, the same number of staff are assigned to their roles day-in and day-out. Similarly, regardless of inbound communications volume, medical practices will often err in their staffing model by assigning the same number of people to manage the secure, electronic correspondence and the telephones, whether it is, for example, Monday morning when volume it at its peak or a Wednesday, when volume may be at its lowest level.

With a static staffing pattern, the staff are often not able to meet patient demand or provide the infrastructure and support to the physician in a logical, planned approach. Instead, on certain days (and perhaps during specific hours), there are more or fewer staff than are required to adequately provide the infrastructure and support for a streamlined patient flow process. In addition, a static staffing pattern often leads to higher staffing cost. When there is insufficient staffing for the work, a medical practice may incur significant overtime as the existing staff must work longer hours to resolve the gap. If the work overwhelms the staff, regardless of whether overtime must be paid, patient experience surely suffers.

WHEN STAFFING IS STATIC, STAFF ARE NOT ABLE TO MEET PATIENT DEMAND OR PROVIDE THE INFRASTRUCTURE TO SUPPORT THE PHYSICIAN DURING PEAK OR FLUCTUATING WORK LEVELS. BY ADOPTING A VARIABLE STAFFING MODEL INSTEAD, A MORE APPROPRIATE AND LESS COSTLY STAFFING PATTERN CAN BE DEPLOYED.

By adopting a variable staffing model instead of a static model, medical practices can link the appropriate number and type of staff for the work. Many variable staffing strategies are available to medical practices beyond the use of part-time, per-diem, or contract workers. These are summarized in Exhibit 11.1 and further described in the following sections.

EXHIBIT 11.1 STAFFING STRATEGIES TO SUPPORT FLUCTUATING WORK LEVELS

Strategy	Description
Staff assignments by clinic session	Staff are assigned by clinic session based on anticipated work volume, such as encounter volume
Work consolidation	Work consolidated with a limited number of staff, with the others reassigned or scheduled home
Voluntary time off or send-off	Staff volunteer to go home or are scheduled off
Super-trained medical assistants	Staff have an expanded work scope and skills to flexibly manage multiple clinical and business functions
Formal cross-training	Focused cross-training of staff to work during specific peak periods
Nurse leverage	Nurse takes patient history and presents the patient to the physician in a collaborative visit model
Volunteers	Community volunteers augment the role of employed staff for basic functions, such as scanning of medical records

STAFF ASSIGNMENTS BY CLINIC SESSION

In medical practices that have adopted a staff-per-clinic-session strategy, a supervisor reviews the appointment schedule, projected same-day patient requests, anticipated communications, and staffing needs to support telemedicine. He or she determines the staffing assignments required for an individual clinic session based on the anticipated work volume and type. The staffing assignments thus change daily depending on the work variation.

WORK CONSOLIDATION

In this strategy, work is consolidated with a select number of staff, thereby achieving economies of scale and scope, improved work efficiency, and enhanced knowledge. Common scenarios for this model include:

- Designation of a nurse unit to manage patient triage and advice exclusively, leaving the remainder of the clinical team to assist the physician with patients in the office,
- Consolidating the work related to care or panel management under a single employee or within a single unit, and
- Formation of a designated call center to manage inbound communications.

VOLUNTARY TIME OFF OR SEND-OFF

In medical practices with a time-off or send-off strategy, the supervisor or practice executive determines the staff required to manage the work for the remainder of the day (such as from 1:00 p.m. until closing) and asks for volunteers to go home. If no volunteers emerge, the manager selects staff to send home due to low work volume.

SUPER-TRAINED MEDICAL ASSISTANTS

Some medical practices employ staff who are trained in both front office and medical assisting. With this expanded skill mix, staff are capable of performing both of these key functions in the medical practice.[1] In this model, medical assistants receive expanded training in front office operations.

These staff perform an expanded range of work functions to include the traditional work of a medical assistant (such as retrieving and rooming patients and taking vital signs), as well as front office work (such as managing inbound telephones calls, conducting patient check-in and check-out, and coordinating referrals), and they may also function in other roles. This staffing model replaces the traditional model where medical assistants, receptionists, and other employees work in specific silos. Instead, "super-trained" medical assistants conduct multiple roles, demonstrating an expanded breadth and scope of responsibility.

With this strategy, the staff can be deployed consistent with work fluctuations, rather than be situated in one functional role where they may have idle time or capacity. In some cases, this also permits the staff member to shadow the patient through each step of the patient visit, limiting the handoffs of the patient from one staff member to the next.

The *advantages* of this model include:

- Flexibility to assign staff based on variable work levels,

- Ability to fully delegate tasks from the physician to the staff, and

- Ability to recruit and retain high-performing staff who have expanded work variety and are active and contributing members of the care team.

The *disadvantages* of this model include:

- Training costs associated with front office operations,

- Potential loss of accountability for a work scope (which can be overcome by establishing standard work processes), and

- Potential limitations on scope of practice of this role, typically governed by the state.

FORMAL CROSS-TRAINING

A formal cross-training program permits staff to assume additional roles and responsibilities during high peak demand, yet the additional work assignment for the staff has some permanency.

For example, a medical assistant is educated and trained to schedule appointments to ensure coverage. On Monday morning during peak call volume, the medical assistant rotates to appointment scheduling. In this fashion, the staff are not merely "helping out," but instead, have this as a defined role and responsibility for which they are held accountable.

Staffing to Optimize Facility Utilization

The only revenue-producing space in a medical practice are the exam rooms and procedure rooms, thus any opportunity to transition non-clinical space into clinical space or to reduce overall square footage altogether makes a positive impact on the bottom line. As we discuss earlier in this chapter, one of the benefits of teleworking is that it permits a medical practice to either reduce its facility size or potentially convert non-clinical space to clinical space.

If a medical practice eliminates the sequential process for patient flow, for example, the separate steps of check-in, retrieval, rooming, visit, and check-out, it can reduce the size of its medical practice facility. Rather than ask patients to travel to the work (for example, walk from the check-in desk to the exam room to the check-out desk), the medical practice brings the work to the patient in the exam room and eliminates the space needed for these functions — and reduces the queuing and wait time for patients when they present to the medical practice.

Eliminate Patient Check-in

Many medical practices have eliminated the traditional check-in area — and its associated staffing — by performing business preparation for the visit before the patient presents to the office or automating the process via a tablet or kiosk. If pre-visit functions have been fully performed, the activity required at check-in is to verify demographic and insurance information in the event a change has recently occurred, obtain waivers and other signatures, and collect time-of-service payments. These functions can be performed in the exam room by support staff, upon rooming. Alternatively, the patient can perform these functions at a kiosk located at the entrance to the practice, or via assistance by a staff member managing the distribution of tablets. A feature now commonly available, real-time eligibility, facilitates the insurance confirmation process. Innovative strategies such as biometric identification (for example, the patient's palm print activates the check-in process) add to the possibilities.

Some medical practices have taken this concept further and have eliminated the waiting room or reception area altogether, with patients escorted to the exam rooms immediately upon arrival, conducting check-in functions in the exam room. In addition to administrative tasks, other practices have integrated medical, social, and family history into the workflow, thus shortening the clinical intake process as well. These ideas become reality once workflow and technology support the historically labor-intensive check-in process.

ELIMINATE PATIENT CHECK-OUT

Other medical practices have eliminated the traditional check-out area — and its associated staffing. The patient's post-visit needs are managed in the exam room by a staff member. This advances the patients' experience, because patients can be serviced without transferring information from one party to the next (which can lead to confusion and even mistakes). Furthermore, patients no longer must wait in line at the check-out area; they are serviced in the exam room from where they depart.

This new workflow is facilitated by recording the follow-up instructions for the patient in the EHR system. If there is insufficient exam room space to eliminate check-out altogether (for example, if leaving a patient in the exam room after the encounter delays rooming of the next patient), the check-out process can be streamlined to allow for automated recalls and referrals to be managed with the patient via telephone or secure messaging after the visit.

ELIMINATE BOTH CHECK-IN AND CHECK-OUT

Still other medical practices have eliminated both the patient check-in and check-out areas altogether. They conduct all clinical and administrative functions in the exam room, thereby altering their staffing deployment model for the front office.

Either change — eliminating the patient check-in area or removing the check-out area (or both) — will alter the patient flow process and, consequently, the staffing model of a medical practice. These alterations are consistent with new staffing models that feature staff who are trained and capable of handling both clinical and administrative roles.

ADOPT A SHIFT SCHEDULE

Some medical practices have extended their patient access hours and improved their facility utilization by running a shift schedule. One set of physicians and support staff work from 7:00 a.m. to 2:00 p.m., for example, with another set working from 2:00 p.m. to 9:00 p.m. The 1:00 to 2:00 p.m.

hour may be used as a wind-down and start-up time for the teams so that each seven-hour block is fully productive. Others may have a traditional business day, with physicians and staff working from 8:00 a.m. to 5:00 p.m., for example, with a separate evening shift working from 5:00 p.m. to 8:00 p.m.

> THE DUAL-SHIFT MODEL OF CARE AND ITS ASSOCIATED STAFFING PATTERN INCREASES PATIENT ACCESS AND FACILITY UTILIZATION AND SPREADS THE COST OVER MORE PATIENTS, THEREBY REDUCING COST PER VISIT.

Patients, particularly those who are time-starved, appreciate expanded access to care. Each medical practice is essentially paying for its space on a full-time basis, 24 hours per day, seven days per week, however utilizing it only a fraction of that time. The shift model of care and its associated staffing pattern increases patient access and facility utilization, thereby reducing the cost per visit, with the high fixed costs associated with the space spread over more patients.

WORK SEGMENTATION STRATEGIES

There are times when a medical practice simply cannot afford to hire the number of staff required for the work or is short-staffed despite its best planning efforts. Situations may also arise when staff have been delegated a high volume of work tasks but find it hard to prioritize their time to attend to each task. In these circumstances, consider segmenting staff time to each delegated task to ensure that attention and expertise are paid to the work.

- *Work Segmentation by Day.* In this model, the staff member is presented with a schedule of tasks and a time allocation to perform each task. For example, a staff member who is tasked with conducting payment posting, account follow-up, credit balance resolution, and denial management may work under a segmentation strategy to focus energy and attention to each of these tasks. A schedule is developed, and the staff is asked to work on a designated task during a specific time slot, such as the schedule depicted in Exhibit 11.2.

Exhibit 11.2 Work Segmentation by Day

	Task Assignment 8:00-12:00 noon	Task Assignment 1:00 to 5:00 p.m.
Monday	Insurance Follow-up	1:00-2:00 Posting 2:00-5:00 Credits
Tuesday	Insurance Follow-up	1:00-2:00 Posting 2:00-5:00 Credits
Wednesday	Denial Management	1:00-2:00 Posting 2:00-5:00 Patient Follow-up
Thursday	Insurance Follow-up	1:00-2:00 Posting 2:00-5:00 Patient Follow-up
Friday	Denial Management	1:00-2:00 Posting 2:00-5:00 Patient Follow-up

The designated hours assigned for each task depends on the work volume and complexity. Use the staff productivity workload ranges previously discussed in this book, blended with the historical experience related to these tasks in the practice, to identify the amount of time to allocate to each task.

- *Work Segmentation by Task.* Another way to segment work is to delegate it in manageable chunks rather than assigning a full scope of work to a staff member. As examples:

  - A medical practice has a shortage of insurance account follow-up staff. It trains a staff member to work a specific type of claim denial utilizing a precise, defined work process. It delegates only those distinct accounts to the staff member to work. In this fashion, a team member steps in to carry out work functions without needing the full scope of knowledge of a business office employee.

⊚ The state's Medicaid database needs to be queried for each of the practice's self-pay accounts on a weekly basis. A staff member is trained to perform this weekly Medicaid "sweep" to assist the business office in the case of a staffing challenge.

By segmenting the work and training just for that segment, some of the work can be delegated and managed during an unplanned staff shortage.

WORK EXTENSION STRATEGIES

Some medical practices have decreased their staffing levels by asking current staff to take on additional responsibilities.

The advantages of this approach are many:

- The best and the brightest staff often can assume added responsibilities and accountability, thus enhancing their professional development,

- If applicable, by paying them additional compensation or bonuses, staff can be recognized for this expanded work scope,

- The staff who are delegated increased responsibility often have a sense of loyalty and engagement with the medical practice above that of a traditional salaried employee, and

- Many take ownership in the work and recognize their role as a partner in the practice and as an integral member of the care team.

Two examples of work extension strategies follow:

- *Medical assistant rooms for two physicians.* One medical assistant rooms patients for two physicians, with one nurse on the phone. In this model, the medical assistant extends his or her scope from one to two physicians. He or she is rooming and anticipating the physicians' needs. In this model, there is often a lag start and end time for the physicians so that the flow of patients throughout the facility can occur in a more streamlined fashion.

- *Biller expands scope of his or her work.* A billing representative working insurance account follow-up is asked to extend the scope of his or her work by also managing remittances and working claim denials. In this fashion, the staff member exercises the full scope of work involved in identifying the reasons for zero payment or under-level payments. Accountability rests fully with this staff member to manage reimbursement from the payers.

WORK ROTATION STRATEGIES

Work rotation strategies are a great way to ensure that staff have the skills and knowledge to perform multiple tasks throughout the practice. Work rotation involves identifying specific days or sessions per day during which the staff member engages in one type of work; other days or sessions are devoted to a different type of work.

Examples of work rotation include:

- *Nurses rotate as care manager.* Nurses are asked to rotate on a weekly basis to fill the role of care manager for the practice's patient population. The registry allows the nurse to determine and prioritize patients, corresponding tasks and communications. The advantage of rotating this role is that it permits focus on the function, and each nurse gains insight into the challenges of patient care that takes place between scheduled appointments.

- *Nurses rotate on flow and telephones.* One nurse is assigned to manage inbound communications (telephones and secure messaging) and one nurse is assigned to in-person patient flow. In the afternoon, these nurses switch roles. Rather than rotate the work by half-day, another option is to rotate the work by day, week or even month.

- *Nurses rotate weekly tasks.* Nurses rotate to work weekly assigned tasks, such as managing post-discharge communication with patients, pulling and processing referrals from the health information exchange, and performing basic phlebotomy functions for the in-house CLIA-waived laboratory.

- ***Staff rotate to manage the front office.*** When patients queue up at the front office, a message is sent to another staff member who arrives at the front office and opens up another station for check-in. In this fashion, the additional check-in staff member rotates into the work throughout the day based on workload fluctuation.

SUMMARY

In this chapter, we draw attention to the important role that part-time, per-diem, contract, and remote employees can play in a medical practice. We also discuss approaches to match staffing with the work, particularly during times of work volume fluctuations and employee absences. As an industry, healthcare has been late in taking advantage of alternative work arrangements. However, given the nature of fluctuating work volumes, combined with the complexity of the work environment, flexible staffing is becoming vital to medical practice success.

ENDNOTES

1 "University of Utah Health Care Community Clinics' Care by Design™, which features the Care Team Model, Appropriate Access and Planned Care." AHRQ Transforming Primary Care Grant. https://www.ahrq.gov/sites/default/files/wysiwyg/professionals/systems/primary-care/tpc/tpc-profile-magill.pdf. Accessed October 3, 2017.

PART 5

HOW TO CREATE A HIGH-PERFORMING CARE TEAM

CHAPTER 12

HIGH-PERFORMING
CARE TEAMS

In healthcare, a patient-centered care team is a prerequisite for success. Medical practices grapple not only with the complex human biological form, but also with the behavioral and emotional elements associated with health and healing. This requires a well-orchestrated approach to each facet of the patient flow process. It also necessitates compassion and empathy. It is no longer adequate for a patient to be treated as if he or she is just a diagnosis or patient number 152 of the day. As you redesign your care team, ensure that the patient is at the center of your care processes.

In addition, a high-performing care team is needed to manage the healthcare needs of a patient population, with each team member fully deployed and engaged.

In this chapter, we:

- Define a high-performing care team
- Emphasize patient-centered work
- Recognize the "care" in care team
- Review steps to create a high-performing care team

WHAT IS A HIGH-PERFORMING CARE TEAM?

The traditional staffing model in a medical practice places the physician at the center of the activity, with each staff member revolving around this core expected to operate in a well-coordinated fashion. However, this is not the reality for most medical practices. Instead of a well-coordinated team, we often witness turf battles between the front and back offices, misunderstandings regarding roles and responsibilities, and some staff who work hard while others shirk their duties. The telephones are ringing off the hook; there is paper, paper, and more paper everywhere (even though we are supposedly "paperless"); computers are constantly frozen or off-line; communication channels and avenues are simultaneous and often loud; the pace is hectic, and everyone is stressed to the max — only to go home and wake up the next day and do it all over again.

> IMAGINE A NEW STRATEGY WITH THE PATIENT AT THE CENTER OF THE CARE TEAM.

By contrast, a high-performing team in a medical practice places the patient at the center of the team (Exhibit 12.1). Rather than staffing each physician, a care team model is embraced. Work processes are designed and executed from the patient's perspective. Once the processes are patient-centric, a physician-led, well-coordinated care team ensures that care is coordinated and executed, and the patient becomes a partner with their care team in their health and wellness.

In a high-performing care team:

- Support staff are highly functional and integrated, with well-rehearsed and orchestrated roles and assignments.
- Process and patient handoffs, from one task to the next, are minimized.
- Patient wait time — for access, information, and visit — is minimized.

In short, the physician leads a highly functional and well-coordinated care team that is whole-heartedly focused on patient access, care and support.

Importantly, in today's medical practices, the care team is often asked to extend across the continuum of care. For example, a care manager may work with a patient to facilitate transitions of care from primary care to specialty care to hospital care to home care. Thus, members of the care team need to not only be internally focused on patients, colleagues, and co-workers, but also need to be externally focused on the delivery system itself.

EXHIBIT 12.1 PATIENT-FOCUSED HIGH-PERFORMING TEAM

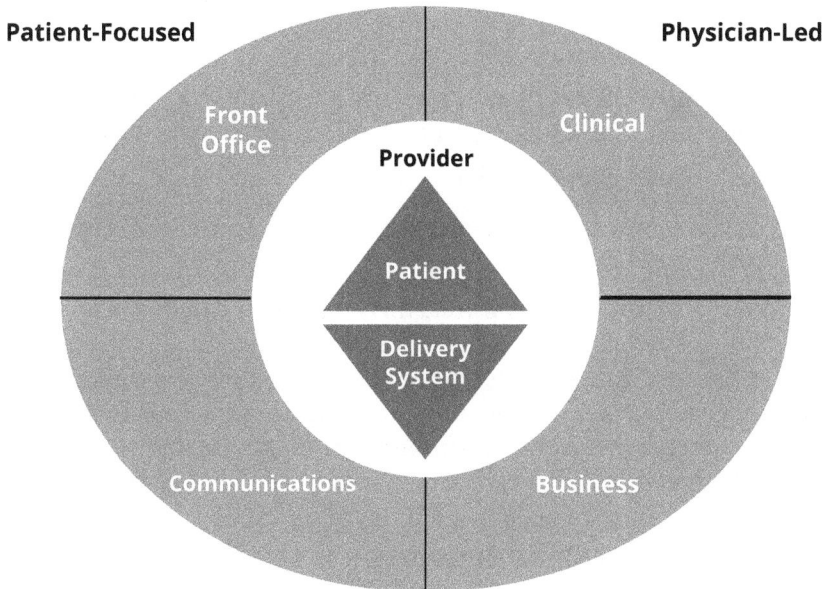

Patient-Focused   **Physician-Led**

Front Office

Clinical

Provider

Patient

Delivery System

Communications

Business

**Each member of the care team coordinates
to deliver personalized care and service**

THE "CARE" IN CARE TEAMS

One expectation for a care team is to have staff who truly care. Patients expect to be treated with compassion and empathy. Yet, we have often run into staff who are neither compassionate nor empathetic. Instead, these staff are "me" oriented and appear unable to extend warmth and caring. You have probably met one or more of these staff members at some point in your career — or have encountered one as a patient yourself.

There are many examples of problematic behavioral styles; here are just a few:

- *It's all about me* — the work revolves around the employee.
- The employee acts as though the patients are a personal interruption, rather than welcomed and received in the practice.

- The patient is treated as if he or she is a number or a disease, not a person.

- The employee tells patients what can't be done rather than what can be done.

- The employee always has an excuse when patients complain about his or her service.

- The employee is not a morning person.

- The employee is not customer-friendly, in fact, he or she is not even people-friendly.

Staff who are not able to demonstrate this most basic of human emotions — empathy — for patients have no place in a medical practice. Compassion and empathy are very difficult to teach. Faced with two job applicants, neither of whom possess the requisite knowledge and teamwork skills, it may be necessary to recruit based on culture and behavior and train for the work or task, rather than the other way around.

CREATING A HIGH-PERFORMING CARE TEAM

Teamwork results from institutionalizing the values of the medical practice, developing clear performance expectations, providing training and development opportunities, and offering ongoing assessment of behavior in the context of the medical practice's expectations. Teaming for effective care management is a core competency of better-performing medical practices.

The following actions can help create a high-performing care team for your medical practice:

- Hire staff based on teamwork,

- Articulate teamwork expectations,

- Evaluate staff on teamwork,

- Share information and expect contribution, and

- Model teamwork behaviors.

> TEAMING FOR EFFECTIVE CARE MANAGEMENT IS A CORE COMPETENCY OF BETTER-PERFORMING MEDICAL PRACTICES.

Hire Staff Based on Teamwork

The reality is that there are team players — and those who are out to operate for themselves. Emphasize teamwork in your job postings, and vet applications carefully. Check references thoroughly, to include specifics on the applicant's experience as a team member. Hiring team players advances your ability to create a culture of teamwork.

Articulate Teamwork Expectations

Define the type of teamwork behaviors you expect in your medical practice. Team behaviors that are often articulated in a medical practice include:[1]

- Meets and exceeds patient expectations for care and service,
- Exercises good judgment and initiative,
- Actively participates on the team,
- Works with others to achieve consensus,
- Contributes knowledge to the team,
- Conducts objective problem-solving,
- Demonstrates interpersonal effectiveness,
- Supports other team members,
- Fosters trust and respect,
- Develops mutual accountability for the work,
- Is creative and innovative, and
- Is positive, with high energy and engagement.

Evaluate Staff on Teamwork

Once you have developed teamwork expectations, ask the staff to evaluate themselves regarding each of these attributes as part of a self-assessment. The supervisor or manager should then provide perspective regarding the staff member's strengths and areas of opportunity to improve team-oriented behaviors.

To ensure that staff are focused on teamwork and to reinforce that you truly expect team-oriented performance, ensure the talent management process and any incentive or bonus plans that are developed for your medical practice focus on teamwork. See examples of teamwork evaluation in Chapter 13: Staff Recruitment, Retention and Talent Management.

> THROUGH THESE ACTIONS, STAFF TRANSITION FROM EMPLOYEE TO COLLABORATIVE PARTNER, ONE WHO HAS A SENSE OF OWNERSHIP AND PRIDE IN THE WORK AND MAKES A TRUE CONTRIBUTION TO THE TEAM.

SHARE INFORMATION AND EXPECT CONTRIBUTION

The best person to recommend a change to work functions and tasks is the person who has been performing those duties, often for many years, and is closest to and owns the process.

Share as much financial and operational information as possible with your team. This includes educating staff to the changing healthcare environment and seeking their assistance in continually scanning the environment, both the external market (to learn about changes in the community, for example), and the internal setting (for example, their own workload and work processes).

Help your staff understand the entire patient flow process — involving both clinical and administrative work processes — not just their specific roles and responsibilities. As examples:

- Require schedulers who obtain patient demographic and insurance information to become familiar with claim denials so that they understand what happens with the information they are asked to collect and verify.

- Ask the receptionist who is assigned to collect time-of-service payments to sit with a team member in the business office who is attempting to conduct self-pay account follow-up to understand the impact of the work when patients do not pay at the point of care.

- Introduce staff members in the call center to the practice suite and ask them to shadow the nurse or medical assistant to understand their world — and vice versa — so that each can understand the impact of their work on their team member.

In this fashion, a more integrated care team is fostered.

Share performance results with staff. For example, staff members who are assigned to conduct insurance account follow-up should know their days in receivables outstanding, their accounts receivable greater than 90 days, and their net collection rate, as well as the targets and goals that are expected of their performance. In this fashion, team members can self-manage and initiate corrections, as appropriate.

> SHARE AS MUCH FINANCIAL AND OPERATIONAL INFORMATION AS POSSIBLE WITH YOUR TEAM AND SOLICIT THEIR IDEAS AND CONTRIBUTIONS.

Let staff know that you do expect them to raise issues and concerns, but at the same time, you expect them to share their talent and recommend solutions to problems. In this fashion, your staff become active contributors to the medical practice. Through these actions, staff transition from employee to collaborative partner, one who has a sense of ownership and pride in the work and work product and makes a true contribution to the team.

MODEL TEAMWORK BEHAVIORS

Ask physicians, practice leaders, and supervisors to model teamwork behaviors. Examples of modeling teamwork include:

- Hold same-day huddles with the staff to review the day and discuss what worked and what did not work from the prior day (or morning session),

- Share practice data and information and ask staff for their ideas and feedback for improvement and innovation,

- Stay calm and exercise a focused determination on improving patient health and wellness,

- Treat every person on the care team as an equal; no one person or one type of staff should be viewed as more important than another,

- Expect more from staff; challenge staff to think critically and assign work to staff that stretches their comfort zones, and

- Take the extra few seconds to recognize the efforts of colleagues in the workplace. For example, say "please," "thank you," and "good work."

Summary

In this chapter, we share the definition of a patient-centered, physician-led team. We also review actions that can be taken to create and strengthen your care team. By adopting specific actions and tools, a medical practice encourages staff to transition from employee to collaborative partner and become active, contributing members of the team. This is not a panacea. That is, you will still have days when things don't go as expected and you will still have staff who at times exhibit outlier behavior. However, these tools help begin the difficult process of transforming the culture of your medical practice to one that values teamwork and staff contribution.

Endnotes

1 Walker, Deborah. 1999. "Laying the Foundation for Continual Change: Teaming for Innovation," pp. 19-30. In Key, M.K.: Managing Change in Healthcare: Innovative Solutions for People-Based Organizations. New York: Healthcare Financial Management Association, McGraw-Hill. Adapted from Team Self-Assessment Instrument, p. 29.

CHAPTER 13

STAFF RECRUITMENT, RETENTION, AND TALENT MANAGEMENT

The intellectual capital required for a successful medical practice rests with your staff. Policy and procedure manuals may provide guidance, but they do not detail how to build a call schedule, perform nurse triage, or determine and collect a patient's unmet deductible. The core competencies of your medical practice are the unique assets of your physicians, advanced practice providers, and staff.

In this chapter, we discuss:

- Staff recruitment strategies,
- Staff retention strategies, and
- Talent management.

STAFF RECRUITMENT STRATEGIES

Be sure to revisit your staffing model each time you have a staff vacancy. It may be that a new staff member is not truly needed; instead, a change to your staffing model may be warranted.

Prior to updating the employee's job description and posting the job vacancy, ask the following questions:

- What functions and tasks have been delegated to this staff member?

- Is there a specific licensure, credentialing, or skill that is needed to perform this work?

- Do we need to recruit for this position or is there a different staffing deployment model that we can use in our medical practice to accomplish this work?

- As part of this recruitment, can we combine roles and responsibilities in new and different ways, thereby elevating or growing a staff member to this role?

- Does the work need to be conducted in the way we have always done it, or is there a new or more innovative way to complete the work that may change our staffing needs?

- Is there a better way to accomplish the work responsibilities, such as outsourcing this role? Is there an opportunity to share this role with another provider or site within our practice?

Through this process you may recognize that many other options are available rather than simply replacing the departing employee with someone with the same job description, skill set, and full-time equivalent (FTE) level.

Let's look at the following example shared with us by a physician who attended one of our seminars. The physician made the decision to fire two under-performing employees. He then convened a meeting with his three remaining employees and laid out two options: 1) recruit to replace the two staff members who were let go, or 2) delegate additional roles and responsibilities to the remaining staff and increase their salaries by distributing the wages of the departing staff to them. Not surprisingly, his staff elected the option of assuming additional work and responsibility with a higher salary. This approach also cost the medical practice less money (due to savings on benefit expenditures), and it helped build a professional care team fully engaged and invested in the success of the practice.

> A STAFF VACANCY IS AN OPPORTUNE TIME TO REVISIT THE STAFFING MODEL. IT MAY BE THAT A NEW STAFF MEMBER IS NOT NEEDED IF A CHANGE IS MADE TO THE EXISTING STAFFING DEPLOYMENT MODEL.

THE HIRING PROCESS

If the decision is made to hire a new staff member, use this opportunity to extend and strengthen your care team.

> NEW EMPLOYEES NEED TO POSSESS THE INTELLECTUAL CAPITAL TO PERFORM THE WORK, AS WELL AS THE RELATIONAL AND SOCIAL CAPITAL TO WORK IN A CARE TEAM PROVIDING SERVICE TO PATIENTS.

Focus on selective recruiting — identifying individuals with skill, talent, and teamwork. It is important to also hire people who take responsibility for their work and contribute to the organization. New employees need to possess the intellectual capital to perform the work, as well as the relational and social capital to work in a care team providing service to patients. Some experts indicate you should emphasize skills and knowledge when you recruit; others profess culture and teamwork. Ideally, you want both.

As a recruiting aid, consider distinguishing your practice from others. As an example, some medical practices not only offer competitive wage rates, but they also extend three weeks of vacation for starting employees (when the more typical vacation offering is two weeks). This extra week of vacation is not a direct out-of-pocket expense, yet it is a great incentive for an applicant to choose your medical practice over others. It also reinforces the perception that you treat employees as professionals (which, of course, they are).

WHERE TO LOOK?

When searching for a new staff member, don't simply rely on one approach. Reach out to several channels concurrently, to include one or more of the following:

- Leading internet job sites,
- Your medical practice website and social networking sites,
- National, state, and local medical associations,
- Specialty societies,
- Journal and newspaper advertisements,
- Technical schools,
- Community colleges and universities,
- Job fairs, and
- Temporary staff agency (with temporary to permanent staffing).

The approach taken by a medical practice varies based on the local job market and the avenues available for communication and distribution of job vacancy information. There is no perfect place to find an employee; seeking candidates via multiple channels is vital to finding the right one.

Despite the multitude of potential channels for candidates, many physicians and practice executives report that their best source of new talent is word of mouth. They communicate job openings to their current physicians, advanced practice providers, and staff. Some medical practices even pay current staff a bonus as a referral fee for a new staff hire (with payment typically made once the new hire has successfully passed the probationary period).

THE INTERVIEW

Once applications are received, conduct a formal review of the applications using a standardized review process. Then decide whether an initial screening by telephone or video will be conducted or whether you wish to schedule a face-to-face interview with each qualified applicant.

Develop standard interview questions and pose the questions to each interviewee. It's important to consult with an attorney familiar with the human resources laws and regulations for your state to determine the appropriateness of your interview questions to ensure compliance with all relevant laws and regulations.

Consider each of the following four areas as you develop your interview questions:

- Specific knowledge and skills,
- Judgment and decision-making abilities,
- Behavioral skills, and
- Teamwork skills.

Open-ended questions elicit more dialogue with the applicant and provide insights into the applicant's teamwork, attitude, and interpersonal style. Examples of open-ended interview questions are provided in Exhibit 13.1.

EXHIBIT 13.1 OPEN-ENDED INTERVIEW QUESTIONS

- What is it about this job that appeals to you?
- What skills do you bring that are unique?
- How would your team members describe your role and contributions?
- What type of work gives you the most joy?

Behavioral questions permit the applicant to demonstrate or explain actions and behaviors he or she would initiate when facing situation-specific challenges. Examples of behavioral interview questions for a medical assistant applicant are provided in Exhibit 13.2.

EXHIBIT 13.2 BEHAVIORAL INTERVIEW QUESTIONS

- Here is a blood pressure cuff. Let's role-play. Pretend I am a patient and please take my blood pressure.
- The patient is confused regarding the medications she is taking. What action would you take to make sure you have the most up-to-date medication list?
- Please walk me through the steps you use to prepare for the patient visit.
- A patient calls to indicate she is not feeling well and wants to speak with her physician. Let's role-play the call and call-messaging.

Determine who will take part in the interview process besides the direct supervisor of the position. If the opportunity allows, convene a small group of staff members to interview the candidate. By having a team involved in the interview process, the medical practice reinforces the importance of collaboration and teamwork — team matters. As noted, be sure to obtain knowledge of laws and regulations that are relevant to the hiring process.

THE ONBOARDING PROCESS

Plan the onboarding process of new staff:

- Develop a formal orientation checklist to ensure that each new staff member receives a complete orientation to the practice and to his or her specific job responsibilities.

- Assign a mentor or teammate to the new staff member so that he or she has someone to approach with day-to-day questions. Ideally, the teammate selected for this role should be a high performer in your medical practice.

- Orient and assess the competency of all new employees on each of your technology systems, to include your electronic health record (EHR) system, practice management system, and telephone system.

- Develop a formal process to oversee the work of new employees, until their competency levels are assessed. For example, the clinical skills of a new nurse should be directly observed. Similarly, a new patient scheduler should be evaluated to ensure competency in scheduling and registration prior to permitting him or her to perform independent work.

STAFF EDUCATION PLAN

Particularly if the local job market does not have a wealth of medical practice operations talent, develop a formal internal education program to train staff and ensure they maintain knowledge currency. Take the following steps when developing a staff education plan.

- Identify national and local resources for each functional area to assist with education and ongoing updates.

- Identify local seminars, webinars, online education, and reading material; engage staff in participating. When a staff member attends a program, ask him or her to bring back key information to share with the team by making a presentation of findings. This also promotes skill development.

- Hold regular staff meetings and ask staff to become experts in assigned areas, such as advanced access scheduling, collections at the time of service, optimization of clinical decision support tools, methods to improve chronic disease management, best practices in patient flow, and other similar important work. Expect staff to expand current knowledge of the medical practice and bring suggestions to change work processes to staff meetings.

- Conduct formal competency assessments of staff; use these to identify additional educational needs.

- Hold dedicated employee development days (or portions of the day) to discuss focused topics. Make sure adult learning is supported; actively engage the staff in the education, rather than use a didactic approach.

Outsourcing

Opportunities to outsource work should be evaluated on a periodic basis, including when there is a staff vacancy. The following work functions are some of the potential candidates for outsourcing in a medical practice.

Revenue Cycle

Vendors can provide the full scope of back-end billing, typically defined as the steps after charge submission. Alternatively, they can perform specific billing functions and tasks. For example:

- *Patient collections.* Collection vendors are now taking on added roles related to patient account follow-up on outstanding patient balances, up to and including the traditional role of following up with patients for delinquent payments. Indeed, some practices have outsourced all patient financial responsibility to a third party, in contrast to managing it in-house.

- *Insurance account follow-up.* Outstanding accounts receivable may be outsourced to a vendor to follow up with payers. Medical practices typically use such vendors as an adjunct to in-house follow-up efforts.

- *Payment posting.* Electronic remittance is increasingly becoming the "norm" from a workflow perspective. The staff in the medical practice are thus freed up to devote their time to examining reimbursement levels and conducting account follow-up rather than simply entering payments into the practice management system.
- *Coding.* Coding vendors provide enhanced coding knowledge specific to each specialty.

INFORMATION TECHNOLOGY

Everything from website management to EHR system support may be outsourced to a vendor serving as a virtual IT department of the medical practice.

ACCOUNTING/PAYROLL

Many medical practices outsource their bookkeeping, accounting and taxation duties to a knowledgeable vendor, freeing up the on-site practice executive for other tasks. Other medical practices partner with a human-resources outsourcing firm or administrative services organization to manage payroll and to pay the appropriate payroll taxes and benefit costs, thereby freeing up financial staff in the medical practice to focus on other areas, such as revenue cycle management.

CREDENTIALING AND CONTRACTING

Most medical practices participate in dozens of health plans, all of which maintain different applications, provider manuals and fee schedules. External parties may be engaged to assist with the initial provider enrollment and credentialing and to maintain the relationship with the health plan as a participating provider. Further, experts may be brought in to formulate the initial contract — or assist with ongoing negotiations of fee schedules and contract terms.

POPULATION HEALTH MANAGEMENT/CARE MANAGEMENT/ COACHING

Vendors are offering a full range of clinical support services, from managing nurse triage calls to conducting care management with a specific patient cohort to working with patients on wellness coaching.

These are just a few examples of the many work functions that can be considered for outsourcing.

STAFF RETENTION STRATEGIES

Competitive wage rates and solid employee benefits are a prerequisite for staff retention. Equally important is the employee's relationship with his or her immediate supervisor and team members. Three staff retention strategies often adopted by medical practices are discussed below. These include 1) career satisfaction assessments, 2) incentive plans and 3) succession planning.

CAREER SATISFACTION ASSESSMENTS

Administer career satisfaction surveys to employees at least once each year. This provides important feedback to leaders to determine if employee needs are being met; furthermore, a survey garners employees' perceptions of their work and work environment. Based on recent research, employees are seeking the following areas in their employment:[1]

- Work-life balance,
- Professional development and growth,
- Advancement opportunity,
- Interesting, purposeful work,
- Opportunity to contribute and provide feedback, and
- Supervisor empathy and support.

Importantly, needs and expectations of employees change over time, consistent with the market and their own individual circumstances. The surveys help in identifying new areas that may require additional focus and attention to retain stellar employees.

An example of a career satisfaction instrument is provided in Exhibit 13.3.

Exhibit 13.3 Career Satisfaction Instrument

Area	Not Satisfied	Satisfied	More Than Satisfied
Assigned work and tasks			
Professional career goals			
Financial rewards			
Nonfinancial rewards			
Communication			
Access to management			
Relationship with supervisor			
Team member interaction			
Work resources and tools			
Continuous learning opportunity			
Balance of work/life			
Care team effectiveness			

What additional tools, resources, and/or support would improve your ability to provide your best work and talent to the care team?

Incentive Plans

Incentive plans are a retention strategy that can be simple, moderate, or complex. The key is to ensure that the development process for the incentive plan is detailed and thorough, and includes examination of any unintended consequences that might arise. Three different types of incentive plans are offered by medical practices, either stand alone or in combination:

- Tangible, monetary rewards
- Tangible, non-monetary rewards
- Non-tangible rewards

> AN INCENTIVE PLAN IS ONLY ONE OF MANY RETENTION STRATEGIES
> THAT CAN BE DESIGNED FOR YOUR PRACTICE'S EMPLOYEES.

TANGIBLE, MONETARY REWARDS

Tangible, monetary rewards are typically detailed in a formal bonus or incentive plan for a medical practice. As examples:

Simple plan: A flat dollar level based on hours worked or percentage of base salary is paid each year as a bonus payment.

Moderate plan: Specific outcomes and targets are identified and, if met, a bonus or incentive is paid to the staff. As an example, staff may share in annual profitability or cost savings associated with staff turnover, reduction in overtime, and other staff expenditures if targets are successfully met.

Complex plan: A complex incentive plan involves multiple targets and goals and may consist of a collection of measures at the individual, team, site, specialty, and/or medical practice level.

TANGIBLE, NONMONETARY REWARDS

Tangible rewards that do not involve a direct monetary payment to the employee fall under the category of tangible, nonmonetary rewards. These rewards often can be described as an added benefit of working in the medical practice. They are different from the traditional benefits of health insurance, disability, retirement, vacation, and sick leave (or paid time off). Exhibit 13.4 provides examples of tangible, nonmonetary rewards.

EXHIBIT 13.4 TANGIBLE, NONMONETARY REWARDS

- Child care services
- Flexible work schedules
- Notes of appreciation (which we tend to find posted in staff cubicles as sources of pride in their work)
- Movie or theater tickets
- Opportunity to work remotely
- Health club membership
- Spa membership
- Aesthetic surgery (one plastic surgery practice offers a free aesthetic procedure each year, up to $5,000 per person)
- Veterinary benefits
- After X years of service, a paid vacation or sabbatical (one practice offers a two-week vacation for two any place in the world after 10 years of service)
- College tuition support
- Masseuse (who comes to the office)
- Dry-cleaning pick-up and delivery
- Automobile cleaning and detailing (while you work)

The four keys to effectively employing tangible, nonmonetary rewards are to ensure:

- Staff understand what they need to do to earn the reward,
- The level of reward is consistent with employees' work and effort,
- Staff value the reward, and
- The administration of the reward is equitable.

INTANGIBLE REWARDS

When we ask why employees love their jobs, we rarely hear them cite their salary. Instead, they describe the intangibles; for example, how well they work with their supervisor or colleagues, their love for patients and the purpose of their work, or the positive environment in which they work.

> PLAN, IMPLEMENT, AND MANAGE THE INTANGIBLE REWARDS IN A MEDICAL PRACTICE AT THE SAME OR EVEN GREATER LEVEL GIVEN TO TANGIBLE AND MONETARY REWARDS.

Intangible rewards often fall into one of three categories: recognition, celebration, and culture.[2] Examples of these types of intangible rewards are provided in Exhibit 13.5. Note that many of these have a strong impact, yet do not have a direct financial cost to the medical practice. For example, changing a job title may have a lot of meaning to a staff member, yet does not need to be accompanied by a salary increase for it to be effective in enhancing recognition of the employee's contribution to the medical practice. Plan, implement, and manage the intangible rewards in a medical practice at the same or even greater level given to tangible and monetary rewards.

EXHIBIT 13.5 INTANGIBLE REWARDS

Category	Activity
Recognition	• Praise • Changing a staff member's job title • Mentorship programs
Celebration	• Social events • Seasonal events
Culture	• Active staff participation • Staff treated as professionals

INCENTIVE PLAN DESIGN

Whether you decide on an incentive plan that is monetary, non-monetary and/or intangible, address the following questions as you design the incentive plan for your medical practice:

- What is the objective? What are you trying to accomplish with the incentive plan?

- Do you want to reward individual performance, team performance, or both?

- Should the plan reward short-term or long-term goals?

- Do you want to provide only tangible rewards or do you need a concerted plan for intangible rewards as well?

- Should the incentive plan be constructed with tangible, monetary rewards or tangible, nonmonetary rewards or both?

- What specific performance should you measure, monitor, and reward?

- Who is eligible to receive the incentive? Should all staff be eligible or only those staff who have met certain criteria, such as years of service or above-average work performance?

- What payment method should be used? Should staff receive a flat dollar amount, a percentage of base salary, a share of profitability related to targets and goals, or some other method?

- When should the awards be given? Should the rewards be granted monthly, quarterly, or at year-end? Will a delay in rewards permit the staff to connect the reward with their performance?

- Should the incentive program be rolled out as a pilot for one year (to ensure it meets its intended goals), or should the plan be put into place with no definable timeline?

- How will you finance the incentive plan? What if you fall short of your goals?

- What are some unintended consequences that you may see with this incentive plan? How will you respond if they emerge?

- Should staff be involved in designing the plan?

- How will you communicate the plan to staff?

Regular review of the goals and performance expectations for the plan is necessary to keep the plan current and to ensure there are no unintended consequences. Most medical practices' priorities change over time, and you want your incentive plans aligned with your medical practice.

SUCCESSION PLANNING

Another staff retention strategy is to adopt a formal succession plan for key positions in the medical practice. A succession plan helps to retain your best and brightest staff while also ensuring continuous staffing of important positions in your practice. High-performing staff are placed on a progressive track for advancement in the practice. Through a combination of mentoring and education to new and/or expanded knowledge and skills, a practice can fill critical staff vacancies from within.

To make sure succession planning works, follow these steps:

1. Identify potential stars — high-performing employees who are also good team players — in the practice.

2. Develop a professional growth plan for these employees that involves additional education and training.

3. Initiate a formal mentoring program to target high-performers and actively manage their trajectory through the organization.

4. Delegate additional breadth and scope of responsibilities to these employees and provide the tools for them to succeed.

5. Work with these employees one-on-one to strengthen their decision-making and cognitive skill sets.

6. Consider assigning these employees project roles to allow them to devote time to expanded breadth and scope of responsibility.

Succession planning can be a win-win for both employees and medical practices. High-performing employees are identified and mentored for advancement, thereby enhancing staff retention; the medical practice is assured of continuous coverage of critical positions in the practice.

TALENT MANAGEMENT

The role of the leader is to keep each individual focused on his or her strengths, helping team members perform at their best. Everyone has weaknesses. If we focus only on the weakness, we fail to capitalize on staff members' strengths.[3] Develop work functions, tasks, and tools that are specific to team members and aligned with their capabilities.

Despite efforts to match talent to the work, at some point during our professional careers, we have all worked with a colleague who is simply not a good fit for the team. In many cases, we walk on eggshells around these employees, trying to avoid them in the interest of office harmony. This approach often backfires as we come to realize that the staff member who behaves badly or acts out is like a virus in the practice, disrupting the best efforts of others, holding back team talent and progress – and, more often than not, causing our stars or higher-performers to seek employment elsewhere. Coincidentally, many of these same employees are often loyal, long-term employees; that adds to the tolerance of their aberrant behavior.

The talent management process of a medical practice encourages us to address the real question we should be asking about these employees: Are they adding value to the practice? If the answer is no, take action consistent with your performance management process.

PERFORMANCE EXPECTATIONS

Articulate the performance expected of staff and expect high levels of talent and contribution as a baseline. For example, in addition to specific skills and knowledge required for a position, most of us want staff to demonstrate the following:

- *Team orientation.* A staff member who is an integral, active part of the care team
- *Continuous improvement.* A staff member who helps redesign processes to eliminate waste and/or improve performance
- *Decision-making and judgment.* A staff member who thinks on his or her feet and makes good decisions
- *Self-management.* A staff member who does not require strict oversight and who demonstrates awareness of self and

understanding of his or her strengths and areas in need of improvement

- *Customer experience.* A staff member who puts patients and referring physicians at ease and provides quality service

- *Communication.* A staff member who demonstrates an effective interpersonal communication style

- *Technology.* A staff member who is facile with electronic tools to aid in efficiency and effectiveness

- *Solution-oriented.* A staff member who provides solutions, not simply points out problems

Develop a formal list of the behaviors and talents that you expect your staff to demonstrate (see Chapter 12, High-Performing Care Teams for additional team attributes). If you do not articulate what is expected, you cannot hold staff accountable. Without an understanding of the expectations, you likely will not get the behaviors and talents you want. The key to talent management is holding individuals accountable for performance and results.

PERFORMANCE EVALUATION

There are many useful resources devoted to staff performance management. In this section, we touch on some key elements to consider when evaluating talent in a medical practice and draw attention to some components that are often overlooked.

METHODS

Define the formal process you will use to conduct staff performance reviews. This process should outline the who, what, when, and how a staff member is evaluated in the medical practice.

- *Top-down:* The traditional method of evaluating employees is top-down. The staff member's direct supervisor prepares the assessment in writing, often using a standard performance evaluation template. The evaluation is then shared with the staff member in a one-on-one meeting, at which time the employee can ask questions or engage in a discussion with the supervisor regarding the assessment.

- ***Top-down and bottom-up.*** Some medical practices ask the staff to review their job descriptions and note their areas of strengths, weaknesses, and accomplishments. The supervisor then meets with the staff to review these self-reported evaluations and provides input. Together, a formal evaluation is prepared.

- ***Physician–administrator.*** Some medical practices ask the physicians for input, with the supervisor combining this information with his or her own to develop a formal evaluation that is reviewed with the staff member.

- ***360-degree assessments.*** Some medical practices have expanded to 360-degree assessment instruments (or a more limited approach). In these practices, colleagues, patients, physicians, and/or staff in other units are asked to provide input regarding the performance of all employees (providers, staff and management) in the medical practice. The supervisor and staff member review this feedback, and together prepare a formal evaluation.

THE KEY TO TALENT MANAGEMENT IS HOLDING INDIVIDUALS ACCOUNTABLE FOR PERFORMANCE AND RESULTS.

COMPONENTS

Regardless of the method that is employed, it is important that the talent management process include:

- Performance expectations of the staff member,
- Assessment of the staff member's performance in relation to the expectations,
- Analysis of strengths,
- Analysis of weaknesses or areas that need improvement,
- Future goals and expectations,
- Staff education and development plan, and
- Feedback from the staff on what they feel they need to do their best work.

This last point — feedback from the staff on what they need from management — is often overlooked by medical practices. The role of management is to provide the tools and support for staff to perform their very best work. The manager's role is to ensure that the staff have the tools and support needed for them to exercise their strengths and ensure that the work is matched to those strengths.

> THE MANAGER'S ROLE IS TO ENSURE THAT THE STAFF HAVE THE TOOLS AND SUPPORT NEEDED FOR THEM TO EXERCISE THEIR STRENGTHS.

PRODUCTIVITY AND PERFORMANCE MEASURES

Assessing the talent of staff in your medical practice not only requires position descriptions that outline expected work functions and tasks, but also the outcomes anticipated of the staff. Use the expected staff productivity ranges that we share in Chapter 4, Staff Productivity to assess work quantity. Coupled with expectations regarding work quality, use these to formulate the basis of performance expectations for the care team.

RATING SCALE AND EXPECTATIONS

A typical rating scale for staff performance includes four levels: (1) unsatisfactory or significantly below standards, (2) improvement needed, (3) satisfactory, and (4) exceeds expectations. Pre-define the specific functions and behaviors required for each of these ratings. Examples of performance required to receive exceeds expectations on a performance evaluation are provided in Exhibit 13.6 for Teamwork and Initiative and in Exhibit 13.7 for Communications Management.

Adopt a similar approach to define the specific performance expectations required of your staff in other areas. There should be no surprises at the time of the performance review. That is, the staff member should have received a) the expected performance expectations and b) continuous feedback regarding his or her performance throughout the year to permit course corrections if needed.

EXHIBIT 13.6 TEAMWORK AND INITIATIVE: PERFORMANCE TO RECEIVE RATING OF "EXCEEDS EXPECTATIONS"

Teamwork and Initiative Performance Expectations	Requirements to Receive Rating of "Exceeds Expectations"
Supports medical practice goals and values	Exemplifies medical practice goals and values through words and actions
Exhibits objectivity and openness to others' viewpoints	Welcomes the opinions and views of others; always maintains a high degree of objectivity
Exhibits tact and consideration	Consistently tactful and considerate in relations with others
Contributes to building a positive team spirit	A leader in building a strong team spirit and identity
Helps teammates when needed	Demonstrates initiative and volunteers immediately when sees that help is needed
Respects others' work time	Consistently aware of unit workload and takes special care not to disrupt others
Makes decisions that reflect a patient-focused care team	Consistently makes decisions of high quality and exercises judgment in support of the patient

Exhibit 13.7 Communications Management: Performance to Receive Rating of "Exceeds Expectations"

Communications Management Performance Expectations	Requirements to Receive Rating of "Exceeds Expectations"
Answers telephone within 3 rings	Consistently treats callers as a priority and demonstrates a high work volume; is extremely efficient and effective at managing inbound telephone inquiries
Uses standard greeting	Consistently uses standard greeting; ensures the greeting is genuinely perceived by the patient
Demonstrates courtesy	Is exceptionally caring, warm and efficient with callers
Demonstrates empathy and concern in call management	Demonstrates empathy, yet responds to callers in an efficient fashion; accurately responds to patient inquiries within work scope
Takes accurate messages	Records exceptionally legible, accurate and complete messages in the patient's record; consistently obtains information needed to facilitate call resolution
Keeps the service promise and practices service recovery	Consistently responds to patients efficiently and effectively; goes the extra mile to recover from service deficits causes by the practice (consistent with established policy)
Exercises judgment in difficult situations	Demonstrates excellent judgment and initiative in managing difficult patients and sensitive situations

By assessing staff talent, work quantity, and work quality, the practice can benefit from the staff member's contribution to the care team — and importantly, the staff member understands the performance that is expected, as depicted in Exhibit 13.8.

EXHIBIT 13.8 STAFF CONTRIBUTION TO THE CARE TEAM

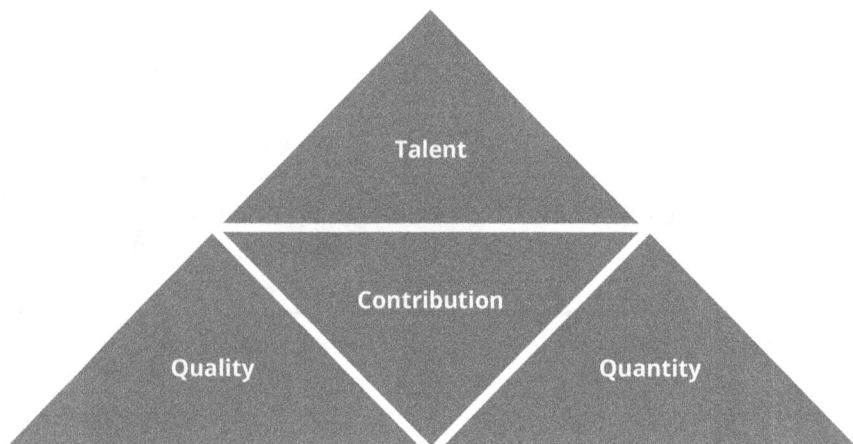

SUMMARY

In this chapter, we discuss staffing recruitment methods to help you identify the right fit for your care team and staff retention strategies to help keep stellar employees on your team. We also address approaches to talent management and the importance of expecting high levels of contribution, holding staff accountable and providing the tools and support for staff to become their best selves. Achieving these goals benefits your staff, your practice — and, ultimately, your patients.

ENDNOTES

1 Ashley Stahl: Employers, Take Note: Here's What Employees Really Want, Forbes, 10/12/2016; accessed at https://www.forbes.com/sites/ashleystahl/2016/10/12/.

Jim Harter and Amy Adkins: Employees Want a Lot More From Their Managers, GALLUP, 4/8/2015; accessed at http://news.gallop.com/businessjournal/182321/.

2 Walker, Deborah L. 1999. "Staff motivation and incentive plan development." Journal of Medical Practice Management. Nov/Dec 15(3):122-126.

3 Peter Drucker stressed the importance of focusing on employee strengths, rather than their weaknesses, and the importance of aligning work consistent with employee strengths. (Per classroom discussion.)

CONCLUSION

The sweeping changes in healthcare directly influence the staffing models embraced by medical practices. We must staff new patient access channels, delivery systems, value-based care models and patient population management. Our employees must master new technologies and learn new knowledge and skills. We must design new staffing models and create a care team that seamlessly works together, innovates, and truly makes a difference in patients' lives.

The following six conventions are continuously addressed throughout this book.

Staff for the Work

The traditional staffing models that assign staff to work with specific physicians or on narrow tasks each day are outdated. In today's medical practice, staff need to be flexibly deployed to manage the work on a given day or a given session per day.

This may include assigning more staff to work the telephones on Monday morning when call volume is the heaviest rather than sustain the high level of staffing required for Monday mornings throughout the workweek. This also includes consolidating scheduling, registration, referral management, communications management, and other similar functions to permit economies of scale and scope. This enables the medical practice to staff for the actual work that needs to be performed; it is not over or under-staffed depending on the day of the week or time of day.

Pull Work into the Practice

Throughout this book, we recommend changes to a staff member's work scope and responsibilities. In many cases, this is to align the staff with the changing reimbursement and delivery system environment. In other cases, it is to create a proactive, systematic approach to the work rather than fix errors on the back end or work in a frenetic fashion.

For example, we advocate conducting patient financial clearance prior to the patient being seen to ensure a clean claim is submitted to the payer and time-of-service payment obligations are met. If this work is not performed before the patient is seen, then staff will need to be deployed in the business office to work claim denials and to follow up with the patient to obtain payment. The determination of when the work is performed needs to be made. The success of the work efforts is higher and the cost to perform the work is lower in the former instance, where the work can be conducted in a proactive and planned approach.

Be Patient-Centered

In this book, we emphasize a patient-centered approach to patient flow. We place the patient at the center of the patient flow process, with a physician-led care team working in coordination to provide value to the patient. This allows us to redesign care processes and redeploy staff to anticipate and meet patients' needs. Importantly, we expand patients' engagement in their health and wellness and meet patients' needs where and when they are expected.

Create a High-Performing Team

We emphasize the importance of teamwork in the medical practice. Given the choice among people, price, place, or product (or, in the case of medical practices, service), it is the people that make a difference in the medical practice. Meeting the healthcare needs of our communities and achieving population health management requires a well-coordinated care team that is both professional and empathic. People are our core competency and it takes a team of dedicated professionals to make a difference in patients' lives.

Expect High Levels of Staff Engagement and Contribution

Your staff have significant strengths and the creativity, innovation, and intellectual capital to help you build an exceptional medical practice. Embrace employees as integral partners in your medical practice, focus on education and training, selective recruitment, and attentive retention. Furthermore, encourage high levels of engagement and contribution by soliciting staff feedback to resolve issues and effect change.

Redesign Staffing to Add Value

Most medical practices have been staffed for episodic visits, rather than value-based care. We encourage you to redesign your staffing model for value-based care. As discussed throughout this book, new roles and responsibilities are required to manage population health, to provide outreach and support to patients, to effectively manage transitions of care, to engage patients in a dialogue regarding their health and wellness via secure messaging and telemedicine, and to ensure that the patient receives the right care at the right time in the right place.

This book presents critical tools and strategies to help you staff your medical practice for value-based care, optimize profitability and performance, recruit and retain high performing staff, and provide stellar patient experience and value.

INDEX

About the Authors

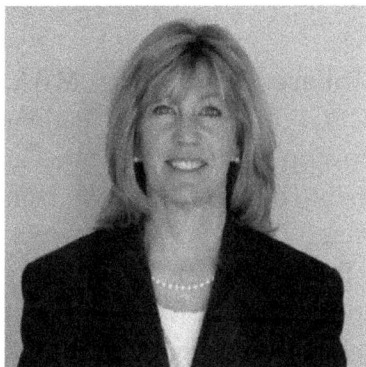

Deborah Walker Keegan, PhD, FACMPE, is a national healthcare business consultant and keynote speaker. She earned her PhD from the Peter F. Drucker Graduate School of Management, Claremont Graduate University, her MBA from the Anderson Graduate School of Management at UCLA, and she is a Certified Medical Practice Executive and a Fellow in the American College of Medical Practice Executives.

Dr. Keegan is President of Medical Practice Dimensions, Inc., and a Principal with Woodcock & Walker Consulting. With rich experience in consulting, education, and industry research, Dr. Keegan brings knowledge, expertise, and solutions to healthcare organizations. She works with organizations to ensure they are relevant and successful today, and importantly, aligned with the changing healthcare environment.

She has co-authored Rightsizing: Appropriate Staffing for Your Medical Practice, The Physician Billing Process (three editions), Physician Compensation Plans: State-of-the-Art Strategies, It's Your Call: Mastering the Telephones in Your Medical Practice, and Patient Access: Tools and Strategies for the Medical Practice. Her presentations and books are rich with "real-life" case material relevant for today's healthcare organizations.

To contact Dr. Keegan or learn more about her services, go to www.deborahwalkerkeegan.com

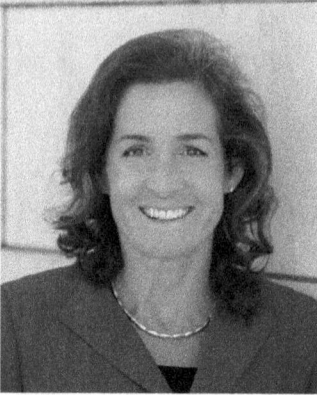

Elizabeth Wallace Woodcock, MBA, FACMPE, CPC, founded the Patient Access Symposium® in 2011. Educated at Duke University (BA) and the Wharton School of Business (MBA), Ms. Woodcock has traveled the country as an industry researcher, operations consultant, and expert presenter. As a principal of Woodcock & Associates, Inc., and Woodcock & Walker Consulting, Ms. Woodcock has focused on medical practice operations throughout her career. She served as the director of knowledge management for Physician Practice, Inc., a consultant with the Medical Group Management Association® (MGMA®) Health Care Consulting Group, group practice services administrator at the University of Virginia Health Services Foundation, and a senior associate at the Advisory Board Company.

Ms. Woodcock is a Certified Medical Practice Executive and a Fellow in the American College of Medical Practice Executives. In addition to co-authoring Operating Policies and Procedures Manual for Medical Practices (four editions) and The Physician Billing Process (three editions), she is the author of Mastering Patient Flow (four editions), Front Office Success, and PCMH and PCSP Policies and Procedures Guidebooks. She is a frequent contributor to national healthcare publications and a sought-after keynote speaker and trainer.

To contact Ms. Woodcock or learn more about her services, go to www. elizabethwoodcock.com.

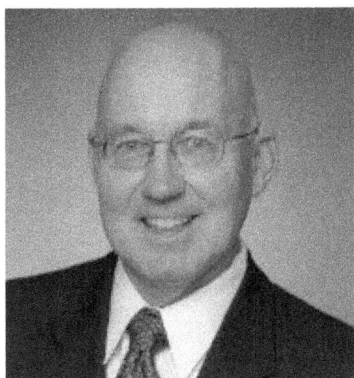

David N. Gans, MSHA, FACMPE. We are pleased to recognize our colleague, David N. Gans as guest co-author of Chapter 2 of this book, entitled "How Staffing Affects Practice Productivity and Performance" and Chapter 3, "Staff Benchmarking." He was also instrumental in providing data insights throughout this book.

Mr. Gans is a Senior Fellow of Industry Affairs at MGMA. He is highly regarded as a national authority on medical practice operations and health systems. He has authored over 125 journal articles, co-authored three books on medical practice management, and was the principal investigator on numerous federal and foundation grants.

Mr. Gans retired from the United States Army Reserve with the grade of Colonel, is a Certified Medical Practice Executive and a Fellow in the American College of Medical Practice Executives.

In addition to his responsibilities for the Medical Group Management Association, Mr. Gans has appointments as a Member, Board of Trustees and Member, Standards and Survey Procedures Committee for the Accreditation Association for Ambulatory Health Care (AAAHC). He is also a member of the Technical Expert Panel, Surveys on Patient Safety Culture, Department of Health and Human Services Agency for Health Research and Quality (AHRQ).

To contact Mr. Gans or learn more about his services, go to dgans@mgma.org.

www.ingramcontent.com/pod-product-compliance
Lightning Source LLC
Chambersburg PA
CBHW060340220326
41598CB00023B/2768